ORANGEVILLE

3 0610 0

Discarded
from the
Library 5

THE
METABOLISM-
BOOST
CLEANSE

D0906032

JAN

THE
METABOLISM-
BOOST
CLEANSE

ROBIN WESTEN

**A 3-DAY DETOX TO
RESET YOUR SYSTEM
FOR MAXIMUM HEALTH,
ENERGY AND FAT BURNING**

Orangeville Public Library
1 Mill Street
Orangeville, ON L9W 2M2
(519) 941-0610

Ulysses Press

Copyright © 2014 Robin Westen. Design and concept © 2014
Ulysses Press and its licensors. All rights reserved. Any unautho-
rized duplication in whole or in part or dissemination of this
edition by any means (including but not limited to photocopying,
electronic devices, digital versions, and the Internet) will be prose-
cuted to the fullest extent of the law.

Published in the U.S. by
ULYSSES PRESS
P.O. Box 3440
Berkeley, CA 94703
www.ulyssespress.com

ISBN: 978-1-61243-361-5
Library of Congress Control Number 2014932307

Acquisitions Editor: Katherine Furman
Managing Editor: Claire Chun
Editor: Lauren Harrison
Proofreader: Renee Rutledge
Front cover design: Rebecca Lown
Interior design and layout: Lindsay Tamura
Indexer: Sayre Van Young

10 9 8 7 6 5 4 3 2 1

Printed in the United States by Bang Printing

Distributed by Publishers Group West

NOTE TO READERS: This book has been written and published strictly for informational and educational purposes only. It
is not intended to serve as medical advice or to be any form of
medical treatment. You should always consult your physician before
altering or changing any aspect of your medical treatment and/or
undertaking a diet regimen, including the guidelines as described
in this book. Do not stop or change any prescription medications
without the guidance and advice of your physician. Any use of the
information in this book is made on the reader's good judgment
after consulting with his or her physician and is the reader's sole
responsibility. This book is not intended to diagnose or treat any
medical condition and is not a substitute for a physician.

To Dr. Bebop

Contents

Introduction

I'm a big fan of cleansing. I've followed dozens of cleansing diets and fasts and written several books about them. Despite the amazing benefits of these cleanses, a few weeks after completing them I noticed that I felt sluggish again. My body was no longer running at the peak performance I had felt while cleansing. What was amiss? Well, after plenty of trial and error, speaking with nutritional experts, and reviewing research, I learned the culprit was my metabolism. It had gone into starvation mode and actually slowed down thanks to my drastic cutback on calories during those cleanses.

I discovered that in order to *burn* calories my body actually *needed* calories. It turns out that metabolism, or how fast the body burns calories, plays a key role in helping us to lose weight and keep our bodies in tiptop shape. The good news? Boosting your metabolism doesn't have to mean intense workouts or a superstrict diet. It does mean, however, making adjustments in your daily life—and it's so worth it.

A quicker metabolism increases your energy through-out the day. You'll feel better, look better, lose weight, and maintain the ability to keep that weight off. And here's a benefit most people don't think about: By simply increasing your metabolism, you'll even burn calories while you're sleeping. With a slow but steady increase in metabolism, it's possible to hit the recommended one to two pounds of weight loss per week. This is the standard safe amount of weight loss recommended by experts, including the Mayo Clinic. Couple this with a cleanse and you're detoxing your body in the process. This win-win combination is what the Metabolism-Boost Cleanse is all about.

In Chapter One you'll learn how your metabolism works. I'll reference several studies proving the importance of accelerating digestion and the downside of a pokey metabolism. Take the quiz, "Measure the Speed of Your Metabolism" at the end of the chapter. Your results will include tips on how you can avoid obstacles along the way as you do the cleanse.

In Chapter Two you'll find seventeen ways to rev up your metabolism, including exercise, sleep, de-stressing and relaxation techniques, massage, sauna sessions, and lots more. Chapter Three follows with a listing of foods that are proven to electrify your metabolism while at the same time cleansing your system. You'll learn that when you eat these recommended foods and combine them with the techniques described in the previous chapter, you'll not only meet your weight loss goal but also look and feel fantastic.

Chapter Four has everything you need to prepare for the Metabolism-Boost Cleanse. This includes a shopping list, scheduling suggestions, and pre-week dietary preparation. At the end of the chapter, go over the checklist: "How Ready Are You for the Metabolism-Boost Cleanse?" You'll find targeted tips depending on your results.

By Chapter Five, you'll be ready to actually do the Metabolism-Boost Cleanse! This section of the book includes three days of breakfast, lunch, snack, and dinner menus, along with a daily schedule that takes you from your waking hours to a deep and renewing sleep.

But that's certainly not the end of the story. Your metabolism can keep on truckin' with the 20 recipes offered in Chapter Six. It's recommended to prepare at least one of these dishes, whether it's a juice, snack, entrée, or dessert, every day.

Of course, food isn't all there is to it. In the final chapter, you'll be given eleven simple steps that will enable you to stay in the metabolic fast lane while limiting toxins, reducing stress, and maintaining your overall well-being. Plus, two additional quizzes zero in on your particular personality type, with tips on how to use your innate tendencies to support your new healthier lifestyle.

If you want to improve your health, feel calmer, look better, and enjoy life to the max, your willpower isn't enough. Wanting it really badly isn't enough. Brute force and sweeping declarations of how positive you are that "this time will be different" aren't enough. What is?

Combine all your positive energy with the steps in *The Metabolism-Boost Cleanse* and you'll be able to take your health and lifestyle to a whole new level.

CHAPTER ONE

What's Your Hurry?

You know the old saying "slow and steady wins the race"? Well, that's good advice if you're a tortoise competing with a hare. But you're not. You're an awesome human being with a desire to be slender, healthy, energetic, gorgeous, and happy. To achieve all these attributes, you need to kick "slow and steady" to the side of the road. Studies show one of the best, and perhaps, only, ways to make it to your goal of losing weight and keeping it off is by putting the proverbial pedal to the metal and boosting your metabolism into super-high gear.

This is especially true if you're one of the 45 million Americans who tried dieting this year and threw away tons of money (according to the Boston Medical Center, in one year we've spent up to $33 billion on weight-loss products in our pursuit of trimmer, fitter bodies) and your results, if any, have been fleeting.

Or let's look at it another way. How come your best friend can stuff her face with sugary cookies, creamy lattes, massive martinis, and greasy pizza and still look like a blade of grass, while you're counting calories and turning down anything remotely delicious, only to find that the scale isn't budging or worse, it's inching up? The answer again: *metabolism*. Your trim pal was probably born lucky and her metabolism is naturally hyper, while yours is set on sluggish. But don't worry. With this cleanse, you needn't accept a genetic fate of fat. The Metabolism-Boost Cleanse will get you going and in a hurry.

Here's a simple biology lesson to explain how it all works.

Metabolism Basics

Metabolism isn't just about your digestive system. It's actually a pretty complex arrangement of chemicals that break down the food you eat; whether it's protein, like a juicy steak; fat, like a pat of butter; or carbohydrates, such as a plate of pasta. In other words, whatever you put in your mouth and then swallow has to go through the metabolic process and be turned into energy.

The key is how quickly your metabolism moves, and that involves a hat trick of factors.

First, metabolic speed depends on how the calories you consume interact with each other. Digesting, absorbing, transporting, and storing your food involves calories. These interactions account for about 10 percent of the calories you use each day. This system, called "food processing," involves a series of complex actions. For example, a study published by the *Netherlands Journal of Medicine* in September 2011 shows there's no metabolic advantage to a low-carbohydrate intake that is independent of a high-protein intake. However, there is a metabolic advantage to a high-protein diet, which will increase the calories you burn by 80 to 100 calories per day. That's why paying attention to what you eat is so important.

Second, your metabolism takes into account the number of calories you burn, whether it's taking place while you're eating, sleeping, or exercising. FYI: You really do burn calories while you sleep, but it has to be a deep sleep. An ample amount of sleep (seven to nine hours) leads to more calories burned both during the day and at night. The bottom line is you need to have a restful sleep in order to burn more calories. Lacking sleep? Well, you'll not only be exhausted, you'll also gain weight.

Third, your genetic makeup comes into play. But don't focus too much on this last point. There are real ways to get your metabolism going even if your family is a bunch of metabolic slow pokes. Besides, your genes only account for around 5 percent of your caloric intake. No biggie.

So, in essence, your metabolism is the sum of all the chemical reactions that go on in your body to give you the energy you need to be alive. But your metabolism doesn't function on its own; it's also controlled by your endocrine and nervous systems. That's why some folks (like your skinny friend sitting across from you with the extra-large fries) have a higher metabolism rate and are able to break down food and sugars faster.

Ultimately, combinations of all the above factors that make up the rate of your metabolism determine the number of calories that you can take in every day without gaining or losing weight. But it doesn't stop there. Two other processes also contribute to your metabolism.

THE TWO ESSENTIAL "ISMS"

Catabolism: This is the process of breaking down things—a series of degradative chemical reactions that break down complex molecules into smaller units, and in most cases releasing energy in the process. It breaks down various types of food into simpler forms that can be used as energy. It includes all those fats, carbohydrates, proteins, and other vitamins and minerals that are found in the things that we eat. This system creates the energy your body needs to perform all its necessary functions. The process is used to heat your body and power your muscles so that everything works just right. By the way: Catabolism is also important for your brain activity.

Anabolism: This is the process of building up things—a succession of chemical reactions that construct or synthesize molecules from smaller components, usually requiring energy in the process. It involves creating energy for the body, but there's a hitch. The energy created from anabolic processes won't be used immediately. Rather, we store it in our bodies for future use. "Store" probably makes you think "fat," but that's not what it's really about. Anabolism keeps your body healthy by encouraging the proper and natural growth of cells. If you didn't have the anabolic process, your body's cells would lose their power and all your tissues and organs would fail and shut down completely. On the other hand, when you take in the proper number of calories and your metabolism is working optimally, anabolism maintains your body's optimum health.

It takes both of these processes together for your body to have the energy it needs. But like everything in life, there's even more to consider.

THE THERMIC EFFECT

The thermic effect of food is the caloric process of digesting and metabolizing different macronutrients in your diet. Keep in mind that there are no hard-and-fast values for the thermic effect of different macronutrients. But here are some generally accepted ratios:

Protein: 20 to 35 percent of calories burned through processing

Carbohydrates: 5 to 15 percent of calories burned through processing

Fats: 0 to 5 percent of calories burned through processing

So what does this mean? Let's say you eat 200 calories worth of protein; your body will use between 40 and 70 of them in digestion. The most common estimate for the total thermic effect of food is around 10 percent of your total caloric intake, but as your protein intake increases, so does this number.

FACTORING IN AGE

Unfortunately, Bette Midler was right when she remarked, "After 30, a body has a mind of its own." If you've noticed your weight has increased every time you blow out another candle, it's no coincidence. Thank your slowing metabolism for this unwanted gift. Beginning as early as around age 25, our metab-olism drags down 5 to 10 percent each decade. That's because total body fat starts to increase, while muscle mass and body water decrease. As a result, you may weigh more as you age, as well as lose some of your youthful muscle tone. Do the math: Without making it your goal to bump up your metabolism, you can lose up to 40 percent of your metabolic power over your lifetime.

The good news? It may be common to gain weight as you get older, but it doesn't have to happen. The Metabolism-Boost Cleanse can put your metabolism back on its youthful fast track.

CHECK OUT YOUR BMR

BMR stands for basal metabolic rate. It's the number of calories you burn daily just to keep your invol-untary body functions, such as your heartbeat, brain function, and digestion, working. BMR is dependent upon your body's composition, which ultimately means the more muscle you have, the more calo-ries you burn every day. That's because muscle is a high-maintenance tissue and requires more calories than fat to sustain itself.

On the other hand, the decline in your muscle mass begins, as you now know, in your twenties, and it's usually coupled with a decrease in your activity level. That's another reason why your waist may be spreading every year and why you need fewer calories than you did when you were worrying about zits. If you're still eating like a teenager and you haven't boosted your metabolism, there's an excellent chance you've been packing on the pounds. The Metabolism-Boost Cleanse can turn this cycle around.

MENOPAUSE

If you've been through it, you already know menopause may mean even more weight gain. When the ovaries stop producing the hormone estrogen, muscle mass lessens to the point of lowering BMR, and when that happens, women can gain a significant amount of fat. Guess where? Your tummy. Belly blubber isn't just unsightly, it also has health consequences. Research shows that if you're shaped like an apple (packing fat in your midsection), you're at greater risk for heart disease than if you're shaped like a pear (gaining weight around your hips and butt). One of the best ways to reduce belly fat is to boost your metabolism. Of course, too much weight *anywhere* will also increase your chances for developing certain cancers and diabetes; it also wreaks havoc on hips and knees.

Despite these influences, remember: A slow metabolism doesn't have to be your destiny. Other factors include:

THE THYROID'S ROLE IN METABOLISM

If you have undiagnosed hypothyroidism (abnormally low activity of the thyroid gland), or you've identified the condition but it's not being adequately treated, almost anything you do to bump up your metabolism has a good chance of going nowhere. So if you suspect your thyroid isn't functioning correctly, your first step should be to get a thyroid test. If you've been tested and your doctor is treating you, be sure that it's exactly what your body needs. This includes the proper drug dosage, as well as supplements to support optimal thyroid function.

Your body's size and composition: The bodies of people who have more muscle burn more calories, even at rest.

Your gender: Men usually have less body fat and more muscle than do women of the same age and weight because they burn more calories.

Your physical activity: 25 percent of your calories go to movement and physical activity.

Cleansing and the Metabolism-Boost Diet

Haylie Pomroy, author of the wildly successful metabolism diet program *The Fast Metabolism Diet,* promises that "you can eat a lot, and still lose weight." We're in Pomroy's corner! But the Metabolism-Boost Cleanse goes one giant step further. While stimulating your metabolism, the Cleanse also encourages your body to say good-bye to toxins, which gives your metabolism an added bump.

Since we're exposed all the time to substances that are bad for us (including pesticides, mercury, and indoor and outdoor pollution, just to name a few), the Metabolism-Boost Cleanse not only kick-starts your metabolism, but also gives your whole body, as well as your mental and emotional states, a brand-new start. It helps all your detoxifying organs—liver, skin, lungs, kidneys, and colon—run at maximum efficiency. It gives any metabolism-related diet added power.

A toxic system is far more vulnerable to disorders ranging from colds, flu, fatigue, and allergies, all the way up to autoimmune conditions, heart disease, and cancer. In other words, a cleanse is the key to overall better health. And, of course, cleansing while boosting your metabolism is the dynamite combo that will not only help you lose weight and keep it off, but balance your mind, body, and spirit.

Wondering just how sluggish your metabolism may be? It's a good idea to get a picture of where you stand before embarking on the Metabolism–Boost Cleanse. This quiz will give a sense of your situation.

WARNING: DON'T SLASH CALORIES!

What?! It's true and here's why: If you cut too many calories, your metabolism will think you're going to starve and it will go into survival mode, putting the brakes on fat burning. The result? Your body ends up conserving energy (calories).

So how do you keep your metabolism pumped while dieting or cleansing?

Answer: Eat enough calories to at least match your resting metabolic rate (RMR). Resting metabolic rate is the energy required by an animal to stay alive with no activity. Therefore, your real metabolic rate is always significantly higher than your RMR. For example, a middle-aged 5'4" woman who weighs around 150 pounds would need to take in 1,330 calories as her resting metabolic rate.

You can calculate your RMR and BMR at www .caloriesperhour.com/index_burn.php.

Quiz: Measure the Speed of Your Metabolism

You pack on pounds much more easily than you can drop them, and diets just don't work well anymore.   ❏ YES   ❏ NO

No matter how much you exercise, you can't lose weight.   ❏ YES   ❏ NO

You gain weight even when you eat very little.   ❏ YES   ❏ NO

Your body is putting on fat in your midsection faster than anywhere else.   ❏ YES   ❏ NO

You've got more cellulite in more places than ever before.   ❏ YES   ❏ NO

Forty percent of women have some cellulite on the backs of their thighs and hips. But if you're starting to notice it on the fronts of your thighs, that's a metabolic red flag.

You're losing your hair and/or your heels are dry.   ❏ YES   ❏ NO

These are signs your thyroid isn't working efficiently.

Your sugar cravings are intense.   ❏ YES   ❏ NO

Since your adrenal glands are responsible for telling your body to release stored fat for fuel, particularly as the afternoon drags on, when that doesn't happen, blood sugar drops and your body signals you to eat something that has quick, easy energy. That usually means grabbing either food with plenty of sugar and/or simple carbs. Good news: Speeding up your metabolism can regulate your blood sugar so you'll have energy all day, without sudden drops.

You feel exhausted.   ❏ YES   ❏ NO

A slow metabolism means that your body is trying hard to use the food you eat as fuel, and this can bring on fatigue. Along with exhaustion, you might also experience general weakness, decreased libido, memory loss, or lack of motivation.

Your skin and nails are damaged.   ❏ YES   ❏ NO

If you have a sluggish metabolism you might have dry, rough, or pale skin. Poor skin, nail, or hair health may also signify a nutritional deficiency.

Your digestion is compromised.   ❏ YES   ❏ NO

If you struggle to properly digest foods, or suffer acid reflux, constipation, or bloating, these may be signs of a sluggish metabolism. Take note: Poor diet can increase these symptoms and slow metabolism further.

You can't bear the cold.   ❏ YES   ❏ NO

Folks with slow metabolisms or thyroid disorders often suffer from poor circulation, making them very temperature sensitive.

Your muscles ache.   ❏ YES   ❏ NO

People with slow metabolisms often suffer from muscle aches or cramps. You may feel as if you have the flu or worked out like crazy even though you've just been lolling around.

You don't have an appetite in   ❏ YES   ❏ NO
the morning.

Don't like to eat breakfast? Chances are your body has adapted to the lack of calories, and it does so by slowing the metabolism.

You're stressed out.   ❏ YES   ❏ NO

Stress can increase your cortisol levels, causing you to overeat and gain weight. The connection? Weight gain causes your metabolism to slow.

You have a hard time sleeping.   ❏ YES   ❏ NO

When your body lacks sleep, it can have a difficult time metabolizing carbohydrates.

You eat a lot of fatty foods.   ❏ YES   ❏ NO

If so, your metabolism is probably slowing down to conserve some of that fat for future use.

You're taking certain meds.   ❏ YES   ❏ NO

Some medications may cause your metabolism to slow and your waistline to expand. Those known to change metabolism in some people include antidepressants, diabetes drugs, steroids, and hormone therapies.

You don't exercise much.   ❏ YES   ❏ NO

When you don't move your body, your metabolism slows down. Consider what happens when you do move: Your heart has to pump harder so that blood can transport the nutrients your muscles need, and when your muscles are working, your metabolism speeds up.

If You Have Fewer Than Two Yes Answers

Hallelujah! Unlike most Americans, you're not doing much to sabotage your metabolism. But that doesn't mean you won't get plenty of benefits from the Metabolism-Boost Cleanse. For one, you'll clear the toxins from your system; for another, you'll jump-start all your body's internal detoxing systems—liver, skin, digestion, and kidneys—and you'll be able to concentrate on healing your emotional life and paying attention to your spiritual growth. As you know, there's always room for improvement. Since you're already ahead of the game, there's a good chance you'll soar into health, well-being, and weight loss. To boost these positive effects:

- ⬆ Set aside at least 20 minutes a day for meditation.

- ⬆ Keep a dream journal.

- ⬆ Commit to being a little easier on yourself. (I know a perfectionist when I see one!)

If You Have Between Three and Six Yes Answers

Take note of those areas where you responded "yes" and analyze whether these are factors you can change, such as eating breakfast, exercising more, or managing stress. On the following pages you'll be given plenty of additional tips on how to make this happen. If your answers are medically focused and include such factors as taking certain medications or suffering with fatigue or muscle weakness, then:

- ⬆ Be clear about what's slowing down your metabolism. If it's medical, make an appointment with your doctor. If the problems are related to your lifestyle, commit to making changes.

🔺 Tune in to your emotional life. You can do this by scheduling 15 minutes of morning meditation, journaling, or taking time for quiet activities, such as walking in nature or working on a hobby.

It is not the strongest of the species that survives, nor the most intelligent that survives. It is the one that is the most adaptable to change.
~ Charles Darwin

If You Have More Than Seven Yes Answers

There's a good chance that if you scored in this category, you have a host of lifestyle habits that are not only keeping your metabolism slow but may also be leading to depression, or at least a lack of energy and enthusiasm. Mark those factors that are holding you back, and when you come across solutions on the following pages, pay special attention to those issues and make a commitment to change.

🔺 Post positive affirmations around your home such as "I can do it!" "I'm going to change my life for the better!" and "I will treat my body and soul right!"

🔺 Ask a supportive friend for help. Sometimes we need help in changing our bad
habits. Also, notice if certain acquaintances
are sabotaging your efforts. Vow to spend
less time with those folks.

CHAPTER TWO

Hop on the Fast Track

Revving up your metabolism isn't just a matter of paying attention to your diet or clearing out toxins. It takes a firm commitment to tweaking certain aspects of your lifestyle. But don't worry; you needn't turn your existence inside out. What's most important about the Metabolism-Boost Cleanse is paying attention to your body, having an open awareness to how you're conducting your life, and then making doable changes to your schedule and your mind-set. Once you get into the Cleanse, you'll be surprised to discover just how naturally these changes become a part of your daily life, how much more time you have than you ever imagined, and how much richer and deeper your experiences can be.

The following factors have been associated with increasing metabolism and/or cleansing. Try as many as you can without making yourself crazy. It's important to stay de-stressed during the Metabolism-Boost Cleanse, so make relaxing into change your number-one priority!

Bad news: 31 million Americans skip breakfast every day!

Feasting at Breakfast

Did you know breakfast is the most important meal of the day? It's especially important when it comes to metabolism. That's because by the time you roll out of bed in the morning, it's probably been between seven to nine hours since your last meal, and your body has gone into starvation mode. At this point, your metabolism is set on a slow pace in its hope to conserve energy. Keeping this in mind, it's not surprising that, according to a study published in the *American Journal of Epidemiology*, volunteers who reported skipping breakfast on a regular basis had 4.5 times the risk of obesity than those who sat down to start their day with food. If you want to supercharge your metabolism, vow to begin your day with a hearty breakfast. The best kind is packed with protein. That's why a good morning menu includes organic eggs.

Nibbling Throughout the Day

Forget about three square meals if you want your metabolism to continue humming steadily all day long. Noshing not only keeps hunger pangs at bay but also helps your blood sugar levels stay steady so your metabolism doesn't spike and crash. What's the magic number of superfood mini-meals? That's up to you, but a standard rule of thumb is no more than 300 calories for each snack. And make each tiny meal a chance to vary and balance your diet to include the proper amount of protein, complex carbohydrates, and healthy fats, as well as important vitamins and minerals. In fact, studies show that people who eat more healthy small meals tend to eat a greater variety of foods and are more likely to meet their daily nutritional needs. Just be sure you don't choose to snack on a big bag of chips.

- - - - - - - - - - - -

Dinner should be your lightest meal of the day. In fact, try not to eat anything after 8 p.m. Some nutritionists suggest nixing food at least 4 hours before your bedtime. This helps your body burn more calories faster and more efficiently.

- - - - - - - - - - - -

Building Muscle

Our muscles make up around 40 percent of our body weight; muscle also contains 50 to 75 percent of all proteins in your body. Plus, muscle is the central tissue for amino acid metabolism and calorie consumption. Now compare muscle to fat tissue, which just hangs out not burning any calories at all. One study published in the *Journal of Applied Physiology* found that older men and women increased their metabolism by as much as 100 calories after only six months of weight lifting. And get this: Strength training raises metabolism long after you're finished working out. Experts estimate that your metabolism stays elevated for up to 39 hours!

How much do you need to pump? It's not only about how many reps you do, but what amount of weight you lift. You might think you should opt for those pretty-in-pink light weights, but research concludes that's not such a hot idea. A study in 2002 by the School of Nursing at Georgia Southern University compared the metabolic profile of women lifting 85 percent of their maximum ability for 8 reps versus 45 percent for 15 reps. The test subjects who were lifting the heavier load for fewer reps burned more energy and had a significantly larger metabolic boost after exercise. So the rule of thumb is: fewer reps +

heavier weights = more metabolic boost. Of course, don't go overboard. Only lift what feels possible without straining.

Getting Cardio and Making It HIIT

Yes, regular cardio like running, walking, and biking increases your rate of metabolism, but once you're done huffing and puffing, your metabolism reverts right back to its regular rate. Not so with high-intensity interval training (HIIT), because it raises your metabolism for several hours after your workout.

HIIT is performed by alternating highly intense bursts of exercise for 30 seconds to a minute ("highly intense" translates into not less than 85 percent of your maximum heart rate) with a slow recovery of one to two minutes. Your metabolism stays triggered after this kind of workout. It's able to do this because your body was put on overdrive, and now it needs to continue to burn calories in order to recover.

You only need to do HIIT for 30 minutes a day, three times a week, or just once during your three-day Metabolism-Boost Cleanse. Here's one way to get going: Run on a treadmill at 9.0 for 30 seconds then walk on a setting of 3.0 for 1 minute. Repeat this 10 times. This takes around 28 minutes total (even including a 5-minute warm-up and 5 minute cooldown).

Those who meditate reduce the likelihood of being hospitalized for coronary disease by 87 percent and the possibility of getting cancer by 55 percent.

Meditating

According to researchers from the Benson-Henry Institute for Mind Body Medicine at Massachusetts General Hospital, a regular meditation practice not only brings you peace of mind, it can also increase your metabolism. The scientists studied 24 participants with no prior meditation practice and another two dozen participants with a minimum of four years practicing meditation. They were tested at the genetic level (via blood tests) both before and after an eight-week program. The researchers discovered a link between the suppression of stress, inflammation, cancer, and trauma with a regular meditation practice. What's more, the scientists also found a positive response for insulin production and an increase in mitochondria, which are the energy-burning centers of our cells. The conclusion? Metabolism increases for people who meditate regularly and it is more pronounced the more experienced a meditator you are.

Ultimately, you want to aim for a daily meditation practice of 30 minutes a day. But if you've never meditated before, begin with five minutes and increase your practice time over a month. You don't need to do anything fancy. Sitting with good posture in a straight-backed chair will work just fine, and simply watching your breath or repeating a mantra like "om" can do the trick. When thoughts come into your mind—and they will—just watch them pass by as if they were clouds floating in the sky.

Practicing Yoga Poses

Sure, yoga is gentle and usually slow, but even so, certain *asanas* (poses) can get your metabolism going because they help the body's cleansing and metabolizing organs work at their highest level.

Twisted Chair: Stand up straight with your feet close together. Bring your hands together with your palms touching in front of the center of your chest. Bend your knees and squat as if you are going to sit down in a chair. Twist your body to the left as you bring your right elbow toward your left knee. Keep your back straight. Hold the position for 30 seconds and then repeat on the other side.

Eagle Pose: This asana requires you to balance on one leg while wrapping your non–standing leg around the standing leg, crossing your arms in front of your body, and sinking your hips back and down, as if you were about to sit in a chair.

Locust Pose: Lie on the floor on an exercise mat or a comfortable rug. Place your arms beside your body with your palms facing the ceiling. Lift your upper body off the floor. Next lift your head back and up toward the ceiling. Then lift your arms and legs upward toward the ceiling, too. When the pose is performed properly, your abdomen will support your body weight and upper thighs. Hold the position for 30 seconds, and then relax your body. Do this exercise three times in a row to boost your metabolism and increase your energy.

Full Boat Pose: This pose will help stimulate your thyroid, which fine tunes your metabolism. Sit on the floor with your legs extended in front of you and your hands resting on the floor, palms down, behind your hips. Point your fingers toward your feet. Keep your back straight. Next, breathe out and then bend your knees and lift your feet off the floor until your thighs are lifted to a 45-degree angle. From there, stretch your arms forward until they are parallel to the floor. Your body should form a "V" shape with your arms straight out from the shoulders so that your hands are at the level of your knees. Hold this pose for up to 20 seconds, and then inhale as you return to a sitting position.

B Vitamins

One of the most important jobs of B-complex vitamins is to work with metabolism. These vitamins metabolize carbohydrates, fats, and proteins and enable our bodies to utilize the energy stored in food. Make sure to get your recommended daily allowance (RDA). Here's how they work:

Vitamin B-1, or thiamine, forms part of the structure that helps break down carbohydrates and fats.

Vitamin B-2, or riboflavin, forms part of the molecule that helps transport energy within cells.

Vitamin B-5, or pantothenic acid, contributes to the structure of several enzymes that metabolize fats, including coenzyme A, which plays a crucial role in the synthesis and breakdown of fatty acids.

CREATIVE WAYS TO GET YOUR RDA

Take it slow: Start by eating one extra fruit or vegetable a day. When you're used to that, add another and keep going.

Be creative: Add finely grated carrots or zucchini to pasta sauce, chili or stew.

Begin the day with veggies: Cross off the croissant and substitute with an onion and mushroom omelet. Add some spice with salsa.

Sip it: A 6-ounce glass of low-sodium vegetable juice gives you a full serving of vegetables.

Roast: Roasting vegees is tasty and simple to prepare. You can use them as a side dish or put them on sandwiches or salads.

Chinese Herbs

According to ancient Chinese medicine, the digestive organs play a role in regulating metabolism by converting food into qi (vital energy, pronounced "chee") energy. If you are not digesting, assimilating, and eliminating properly, you'll have a tough time losing weight and experience many of the symptoms of low thyroid, which includes a slow metabolism. There are several herbs that are useful for restoring a healthy metabolism by improving assimilation and elimination, reducing congestion, breaking down fats and proteins, lubricating and activating the intestines, and keeping the thyroid in tip-top order. When the appropriate herbs are taken for your overall condition, your body becomes more balanced, and weight loss is one of its benefits. But this isn't a one-size-fits-all pre-scription. You'll need to make an appointment with a professional Chinese herbalist to discover if and what herbs your body can use.

Acupuncture

Using acupuncture treatments for metabolism is based on the philosophy that a sluggish metabolism and weight gain may be the result of disturbed energy flow to and from the regulating center of the brain, which is called the hypothalamus. The hypothalamus is responsible for maintaining a balance that allows your body to run in sync. The hypothalamus regu-lates hormones as well as neurochemicals, and helps to control thirst and hunger, as well as temperature and circadian rhythm.

During an acupuncture session, points on the body are chosen for overall well-being with the objective of increasing circulation of the blood and qi and soothing the nervous system. Acupuncture for cleansing, metabolic boost, and weight loss is most effective with a minimum of 10 treatments over a few weeks' time. With some time and patience, you will find that acupuncture and weight loss complement each other well.

Massage

If you book a massage, I recommend a "lymphatic drainage" treatment because it cleanses your organs, speeds up metabolism and leads to deep relaxation. Our lymph is responsible for the ultimate detox system. It delivers nutrients to cells and carries away excess water, cellular waste, bacteria, viruses, and toxins. A therapist trained in lymphatic drainage massage stimulates your lymph system with light, circular pumping movements. By stimulating the lymphatic system, the massage therapist helps drain puffy, swollen tissues, supports the body's immune system, and helps with your body's natural waste removal or detoxification. Manual lymph drainage should have a very soothing, relaxing effect. It can be used as part of a facial, or as a whole body treatment.

Chewing

This is where it all starts, because chewing is the first stage of digestion. Saliva is super important, since it contains alkaline digestive enzymes, essential for digestion. How much should you chew? Well, this depends on opinion. Some chewing enthusiasts suggest doing it until your food turns totally to liquid. They say this will help you digest, assimilate, eliminate, and metabolize most thoroughly. Others say 40 times, no matter what, will do the trick. Chinese researchers reported August 2013 in the *American Journal of Clinical Nutrition* that obese men consumed about 12 percent fewer calories when they chewed each bite 40 times than when they chewed 15 times, and they had lower levels of ghrelin, the so-called hunger hormone produced in the stomach. But don't get hung up on that count. Just paying attention and gaining an awareness of chewing your food will help you slow down, and in the process you'll set the stage for faster metabolism. Like most worthwhile things in life, this takes time to master.

Sweating

Saunas, steam baths, and well-regulated sweat lodges all work by generating heaps of sweat and in the process detoxifying the body and helping to relax your mind. Since your skin is the largest organ in your body, pores play a huge role in cleansing. Sweating transforms toxins from lipid-soluble, or oil-based, forms into water-soluble ones that are easier to eliminate. Then the sweat carries toxins out of the body and flushes them through the pores. Sweating also:

Improves blood circulation: It increases and improves the rate of blood circulation and breathing.

Encourages weight loss: A sauna, for example, is similar to mild exercise because it burns about 300 calories per average session.

Promotes mind relaxation: Saunas and steam rooms are essentially places to relax. Regular sessions help to relieve physical and mental fatigue and stress.

Speeds up metabolism: Heating the tissues in your body puts the mojo on metabolism because your cells become capable of eliminating toxins more effectively.

I'm not out there sweating for three hours every day just to find out what it feels like to sweat.

~ Michael Jordan

Soaking Up Sunshine

Research shows that when you spend lots of time indoors, especially if your environment lacks sunlight, you sleep more, slow down your metabolism, and gain weight. The best time to take advantage of daylight hours are between 11 a.m. and 3 p.m. because your metabolism is most active during this time. So, make it a point during this period to take a brisk walk outside, or at the very least, stand by a window that lets in the sun and bask in the rays.

Standing Up

Something as simple as getting out of your chair and working while standing can have a positive effect on the speed of your metabolism. In one study, researchers discovered that inactivity (4 hours or more) causes a near shutdown in an enzyme that controls fat and cholesterol metabolism. To keep this enzyme active and increase your fat-burning capability, break up long periods of downtime simply by standing up.

Listening to Music

Tune into this: Studies show listening to music can affect your metabolism. According to a report in the journal *Nutrition*, music helps in the regulation of the hypothalamic-pituitary axis, the sympathetic nervous system, and the immune system, which all have key functions in the regulation of metabolism and energy balance. Recent findings also show music affects metabolic recovery from stress, the regulation of gastric and intestinal motility, and the moderation of cancer-related gastrointestinal symptoms, as well as the increase of lipid metabolism and lactic acid clearance, which boosts blood flow to the organs, such as the liver and kidneys, during *and after* exercise, when the body is recovering from exertion.

Turn off the TV! According to research from the University of Vermont, when you cut your television time in half, you'll burn more calories each day.

Deep Breathing

Breathing in deeply draws in more oxygen and allows your body's cells to produce even more energy, and, in the process, increases your rate of metabolism. By thinning your blood, oxygen lowers your blood pressure and blood flows more quickly through your body, which improves your metabolism. The reason? The more oxygen in your body, the faster your metabolism will become. But don't be in too much of a rush. Increasing your lung capacity and achieving deeper breathing takes time, because your body needs to adjust to increased oxygen levels. The secret is to practice daily, patiently, and gradually.

Try this "fire breathing" exercise to improve your metabolism and give you a calm but energized feeling. You can stand or sit for this exercise, but don't lie down. Inhale through your nose for the count of four to fill your lungs completely. Once your lungs feel full, start doing "fire breathing" by taking eight to ten quick tiny breaths, inhaling and exhaling without pausing. Exhale to empty your lungs. Although you'll ultimately want to repeat the exercise for 30 repetitions, begin with a series of 10 on your first day and add breaths each time you practice.

Grabbing More Shut-Eye

When you don't get enough sleep, you throw off your levels of leptin and ghrelin. These are the hormones that help regulate energy use (metabolism) and appetite. Research from both Stanford University and the University of Wisconsin shows that if you only sleep for five hours, your body reduces its level of leptin by 15.5 percent and increases levels of ghrelin by 14.9 percent. What should you do to set your metabolism on high? Researchers say aim for nine hours nightly.

Tough time getting enough sleep? Try these tips:

Avoid caffeine for four to six hours before bedtime: This may be obvious, but too much caffeine right before bedtime will affect your sleep patterns.

Clock your alcohol consumption: Drinking may help bring on sleep, but after a few hours it acts as a stimulant, increasing the number of awakenings and generally decreasing the quality of sleep later in the night. Avoid drinking within three hours of bedtime.

Create a bedroom sleep sanctuary: A quiet, dark, and cool environment promotes sound slumber. Lower the volume of outside noise with earplugs or a "white noise" appliance. Use heavy curtains, blackout shades, or an eye mask to block light, a powerful cue that tells the brain that it's time to wake up. Keep computers, TVs, and work materials out of the room. If your pet regularly wakes you during the night, you may want to consider keeping it out of your bedroom.

Stay cool: Keep your bedroom between 60 and 75°F and make sure it's ventilated.

Create a pre-sleep routine: Ease the transition from wake time to sleep time with a period of relaxing activities an hour or so before bed. Take a bath (the rise, then fall in body temperature promotes drowsiness), read a book, watch television, or practice relaxation exercises. Avoid stressful, stimulating activities, like doing work, discussing emotional issues, or watching adrenaline-charged programs.

Only go to bed when you're really tired: If you're not asleep after 20 minutes, get out of bed, go to another room, and do something relaxing, like reading or listening to music until you are tired enough to sleep.

Hide the clock: Looking at the time, either when you're trying to fall asleep or when you wake in the middle of the night, can actually increase stress, making it harder to fall asleep. Turn your clock's face away from you.

Stick to a schedule: Going to bed and waking up at the same time each day sets the body's "internal clock" to expect sleep at a certain time night after night. Try to stick as closely as possible to your routine on weekends to avoid a Monday morning sleep hangover.

Eat light evening meals: Finish your modest dinner several hours before bedtime, and avoid foods that cause indigestion. If you get hungry at night, snack on foods that (in your experience) won't disturb your sleep, such as dairy foods or carbohydrates.

Exercise early: Yes, exercise promotes restful sleep if it's done several hours before you go to bed. Exercise stimulates the body to secrete the stress hormone cortisol, which helps activate the alerting mechanism in the brain. This is fine, unless you're trying to fall asleep. Try to finish exercising at least four hours before bed, or work out earlier in the day.

The way you think, the way you behave, the way you eat, can influence your life by 30 to 50 years.

~ Deepak Chopra

CHAPTER THREE

Magic Metabolism Foods

It's natural when you're trying to lose weight to fixate on all those so-called bad foods. You know what I'm talking about—a greasy slice of pizza, a superfudge brownie, a bowl of salty chips, or a basket of bread. Those are the kinds of foods we can crave like crazy. But you can avoid the cravings trap. What's the best antidote for feeling that you have to give up the most delicious foods in the world? Learn to embrace what lands on your plate.

On the Metabolism-Boost Cleanse, it's easy to do because there are lots of delicious and healthy food choices available. Don't be surprised if you end up getting totally hooked on green tea, avocado, or oatmeal; it happens. If you waver, remind yourself that you'll not only boost your metabolism, but also burn calories, combat fat, look great, have tons more energy, and feel lots happier. It may sound too good to be true, but it's not. Many of the foods described in this chapter not only increase your metabolism and trigger hormones that release fat, but also help you to eliminate toxins through your organs and tissues, and ultimately help you lose your taste for bad-for-you, fatty junk food.

Are you ready to take a bite or sip of something super healthy? Here are your choices.

Ice Water

Scientists at the University of Utah found that volunteers who drank eight to twelve 8-ounce glasses of water per day had higher metabolic rates than those who downed only four glasses. If you make it ice water, you'll get even more of a metabolic kick. That's because your body burns more calories in order to heat the cold water to your core temperature. In order for cold aqua to leave its water mark, you have to make it a habit and drink at least eight chilly glasses a day.

Chili Peppers

Capsaicin, the compound that makes chili peppers burn your tongue, also puts a fire in your metabolism. According to a study reported in the *Journal of Nutritional Science and Vitaminology,* eating about 1 tablespoon of chopped red or green chilies will ignite your body's heat production by increasing the activity of your sympathetic nervous system (responsible for the fight-or-flight response). The result is a metabolism spike of about 23 percent. It's only temporary, but worth the charge. You can add chilies to pizza, salsa, pastas, and potatoes. FYI: For the adventurous, Dr. Mehmet Oz (cardiothoracic surgeon, author, and television personality) suggests you charge up your metabolism with something spicy first thing in the morning.

Chilies are an intense taste sensation! When capsaicin, the primary substance found in chilies, is ingested, the sensory nerves of the mouth and throat send a message to the brain so that heart rate and sweating automatically increase, and there's also a bump in the body's level of feel-good endorphins.

Iron

Women lose iron during their monthly period, and this loss can interfere with the speed of metabolism. That's because iron helps carry oxygen to your muscles. If your iron levels run too low, your muscles don't get enough CO_2, your energy plummets, and your metabolism gets sluggish. You don't have to take supplements (they can be constipating and no one wants *that*!). Instead, choose iron-fortified cereals, beans, and dark leafy greens like spinach, bok choy, and broccoli.

THREE BIG DOS

Do Go Organic: Organochlorines (chemicals in pesticides) can interfere with your body's energy-burning process and make it harder to lose weight, according to the findings of a Canadian study, published in the *International Journal of Obesity* in July 2004. Researchers found that dieters who ate the most toxins experienced a greater-than-normal dip in metabolism and had a harder time losing weight. That's because pesticides can disrupt mitochondrial activity and thyroid function. Opt for fresh, organic foods whenever possible. And for heaven's sake, avoid heavily processed foods altogether!

Do Eat Plenty of Protein: All foods create a thermic effect and will slightly boost your metabolism. However, eating protein gives your body a bigger metabolic boost than eating carbohydrates or fats because it helps to build and maintain lean muscle mass. And here's the thing: Even at rest, muscle burns more calories than fat. Make sure to incorporate lean protein into most every meal. Best protein sources include fish, chicken breast, turkey breast, lean red meat, skim milk, nonfat yogurt, eggs and egg substitutes, tofu, beans, and lentils.

Do Get Your Fill of Fiber: Fiber can rev your fat burn by as much as 30 percent. Studies find that those who eat the most fiber gain the least weight over time. Aim for about 25 grams a day—the amount in about three servings each of fruits and vegetables.

Omega-3s

Eating plenty of fish rich in omega-3 fatty acids, such as salmon, herring, and tuna, helps to boost metabolism. These kinds of fish balance blood sugar, as well as reduce the body's inflammation. In the process, metabolism is regulated. As a bonus, omega-3s may also affect how quickly fat is burned. According to a study reported in the journal *Obesity Research,* rats that ate large amounts of fish oil when they exercised lost more weight than exercising rats that didn't ingest large doses of the fish oil. How much should you swallow? One thousand to two thousand milligrams a day is usually recommended. If you can't stand the aftertaste, you can try flaxseed oil instead.

Oatmeal

This superfood is rich in fat-soluble fiber, which requires a lot of calories to break down; in the process it gives your metabolism a boost. Eating oatmeal can also help decrease your cholesterol levels and reduce your risk of heart disease. This slow-release carbohydrate also offers long-lasting energy without the spikes associated with sugar-rich foods. What's the big deal with that? You want to keep your insulin levels low, as spikes in this chemical tell the body that it needs to begin storing extra fat.

Grapefruit

Studies indicate that eating grapefruit can reduce insulin levels. Lower insulin levels after meals can help your body process food more quickly and efficiently. This means that you burn more calories and store less fat. Plus, grapefruit contains naringenin, an antioxidant that researchers at the Scripps Clinic in California found helps your body use insulin more efficiently, keeping your blood sugar in check and increasing the number of calories you burn.

Freshly squeezed grapefruit juice that's stored, covered, in the refrigerator will retain 98 percent of its vitamin C for up to a week.

Almonds

Several clinical studies show that almonds, as part of a diet low in saturated fat, can lower cholesterol. These groundbreaking studies show how a handful of almonds a day consistently lowers LDL (bad) cholesterol levels. Plus, almonds make a filling snack; they contain protein, fiber, and monounsaturated fat, all of which may help keep you satisfied. They're also the most nutritionally dense nut, meaning almonds provide the most healthy calories and nutrition for the smallest serving size. One serving of almonds, or about a handful, is an excellent source of vitamin E (an antioxidant) and a good source of fiber, which helps keep you full. Almonds also offer heart-healthy monounsaturated fat.

Apples

That oft-repeated adage "An apple a day keeps the doctor away" is backed up by solid science. Apples are rich in the soluble fiber pectin, which lowers cholesterol and other body fats via several mechanisms. An array of phytochemical antioxidants adds further protection by keeping blood lipids from hardening. What's more, apple antioxidants have an anticancer effect by inhibiting cancer cell proliferation. The greatest concentration of antioxidants is in the peel. An apple's peel contains insoluble fiber, the same fiber found in bran. But the flesh is where the pectin is. Eating an apple each day can also help prevent metabolic syndrome, a disorder associated with abdominal fat, cardiovascular disease, and diabetes.

Apples ripen six to ten times faster at room temperature than if they are refrigerated.

Cinnamon

Did you know that cinnamon is a natural blood sugar stabilizer? A study confirms that a teaspoon of cinnamon added to a dessert helped to temper blood sugar spikes. In fact, researchers are still trying to determine whether cinnamon could be an alternative treatment for type-2 diabetes. That's because cinnamon imitates the biological activity of insulin and increases the metabolism of glucose. Since high blood sugar levels can lead to increased fat storage in the body, cinnamon helps prevent this increased storage of fat and enables you to lose weight. In addition, it influences the manner in which sugar is metabolized by the body and prevents the transformation of the metabolized sugar into fat. Cinnamon also delays the passing of food from the stomach into the intestine. The result? You feel satisfied for a longer time and eat less. And? You lose weight. Plus, cinnamon also helps the body to process carbohydrates more efficiently, which helps you lose those extra pounds. Studies show that abdominal fat is more sensitive to the effects of cinnamon than fat from other parts of the body is.

Olive Oil

Healthy monounsaturated fats like olive oil can actually aid the body in burning calories and bump up your metabolism. In fact, all healthy monounsaturated fats have been shown to burn off three times faster than bad fats, like the trans fats found in commercial food products. Olive oil's fat-fighting benefits are due to the fact that it's rich in oleic acid, a fatty acid that helps fat tissues by stopping them from absorbing fat from blood cells, and further stimulates the secretion of fat cells into the bloodstream so that they can be burned off. Researchers have also shown that taking a spoonful of olive oil at breakfast boosts metabolism by 60 percent. Even so, to get the ultimate benefit, you have to replace other types of fat, like cream or butter, with olive oil, and consume it only in limited quantities.

Avocado

This creamy pale green fruit may be high in fat and calories, but it's also packed with fiber, vitamins, and minerals. More importantly, most of the calories in an avocado come from monounsaturated fats, which help control your metabolic rate. The secret is avocado's rich amount of L-carnitine, an amino acid found in your body's liver that can boost your fat-burning metabolism. It helps to facilitate fat metabolism and promotes fat loss. Additionally, it's known to boost energy production in muscle cells and increase blood circulation in the brain.

Avocados provide all 18 essential amino acids necessary for the body to form a complete protein.

Beans

An ideal source of lean protein, beans are chock-full of both soluble and insoluble fiber, which help lower insulin levels after digestion, causing your body to store less fat. The process of digesting the fiber and proteins in beans burns extra calories, too. The beans with the most protein are fava beans, soybeans, lima beans, black beans, and navy beans.

Brown Rice

The all-important fiber in brown rice and its effects on insulin levels are what make this a great metabolism-boosting food. Choosing a whole, unrefined carb like brown rice instead of white rice, white flour, and other processed carbs promotes weight loss.

Dark Chocolate

Yes! Scientists have discovered that eating dark chocolate can actually aid in weight loss. The benefit comes from chocolate's effect on stress hormones. Study subjects who ate chocolate each day had reduced levels of the stress hormone cortisol, which prompts the body to store fat. And, the *Journal of Proteome Research* reported that dark chocolate actually alters the human metabolism in a good way. The monounsaturated fats in dark chocolate boost your metabolism, which stimulates your body to burn fat. Another added benefit: The smell of chocolate increases theta brain waves, which trigger relaxation.

- - - - - - - - - - - - - - -

All you need is love. But a little chocolate now and then doesn't hurt.
~ Charles M. Schulz

- - - - - - - - - - - - - - -

Gingerroot

Ginger works in a similar way to the capsaicin in hot peppers; the heat of gingerroot can decrease appetite, aid in digestion, and increase metabolic rates after eating. Ginger can help digestion as well increase body temperature and metabolic rates as much as 20 percent after eating. Sliced fresh ginger is excellent in a stir-fry.

Ginger tea is a trusted cold and flu fighter, and assists the body in the removal of excess toxins. It also cleanses the digestive tract and the kidneys, as well as increases circulation by warming the body. Try adding sliced or grated ginger to boiling hot water and steep for five minutes (see page 104 for my favorite Fresh Ginger Tea recipe).

Vinegar

A study of 175 overweight Japanese men and women found that acetic acid in vinegar may "switch on" genes that release proteins that break down fat. The study participants who drank either 1 or 2 tablespoons of apple cider vinegar daily for 12 weeks significantly lowered their body weight, BMI, visceral fat, and waist circumference.

Quinoa

Fairly new on the health scene, this is a terrific metabolic charger because it's a powerful source of protein and fiber. It not only fights off hunger, but also burns fat. You can eat it as part of an entrée or a side dish, or even for breakfast like you would oatmeal. Since it's a seed (not a grain), you can also add it to salads.

Blueberries

Packed with antioxidants, a serving of blueberries each day will rev your metabolism to the max. According to a 2011 study reported in *The American Journal of Clinical Nutrition,* consuming a cup of blueberries per week can lower blood pressure and speed up metabolism due to its high levels of anthocyanins (a type of antioxidant). Another study suggests blueberries can lower levels of LDL (bad) cholesterol, potentially reducing the risk of coronary heart disease. Blueberries may also inhibit the growth of breast cancer cells. It works so well because the oxidation of cells causes your metabolic rate to slow down. So eating more antioxidants like blueberries will interrupt this process and keep your metabolic rate on high.

Chia Seeds

Packed with omega-3 fats, fiber, and protein, these tiny seeds help suppress the appetite, fire up your metabolism, and turn on glucagon, one of the body's fat-burning hormones. The trick is to soak them in water for 15 minutes so they swell up to 10 times their size. The larger the seeds are, the more quickly your stomach will release those hormones that let you know you're feeling full and satisfied.

Coconut Oil

Not all dietary fats are created equal. Coconut oil is rich in medium-chain triglycerides (MCTs), which your body preferentially uses for energy, leaving less opportunity for them to be stored as fat. A study published in the *American Journal of Clinical Nutrition* showed greater abdominal fat loss over a 16-week period when MCTs were consumed versus olive oil. That doesn't mean ditching your olive oil (it has other beneficial properties—see page 51). You may want to consider using coconut oil for cooking and olive oil for a salad dressing.

Eggs

Why eggs? Well they're probably one of the best breakfast foods to help boost your metabolism. Eggs supply your body with the right amount of protein, omega-3 fats, healthy B vitamins, and essential amino acids. Eggs also have iron, which the metabolism needs to function at its best. Multiple studies have shown that the chromium found in eggs is an important mineral for your body and is needed for blood sugar regulation. But just make sure the eggs you eat are organically raised, free of antibiotics, and from free-range chickens.

An egg white is made mainly of a protein called albume, and also contains niacin (vitamin B3), riboflavin (vitamin B2), chlorine, magnesium, potassium, sodium, and sulfur. The white contains about 57 percent of an egg's protein.

Watermelon

According to a study published in the *Journal of Nutrition*, the amino acid arginine, which is abundant in watermelon, can promote weight loss. Researchers supplemented the diets of obese mice with arginine over 3 months and found that it decreased body-fat gains by an impressive 64 percent. Adding this amino acid to the diet enhanced the oxidation of fat and glucose and increased lean muscle, which burns more calories than fat does and increases metabolism.

TWO BIG DON'TS

Don't Consume Trans Fats: Unless you live under a rock, you've heard by now how bad trans fats are for you. But did you know trans fats also slow down your body's ability to burn fat? Trans fats bind to fat and liver cells and slow metabolism. Eating trans fats can also lead to insulin resistance and inflammation, both of which cripple metabolism and can cause weight gain.

Don't Cut Calories Too Much: If you slash too many calories, your body goes into starvation mode and slows down your metabolism. You need to eat enough calories to, at the very least, meet your resting metabolic rate (RMR). That's what you would burn if you just hung out in bed. See page 15 for more on RMR.

CHAPTER FOUR

Prepare to Accelerate

Maybe you've already mastered the basics of eating for a faster metabolism; you're here because you're ready to go one step further and detox your system. Or perhaps this is your first experience with supercharging your metabolism and you're lucky enough to be coupling it with the Metabolism-Boost Cleanse. Either way, it's reason to celebrate—and cause to be realistic.

Unless you prepare well for at least a week in advance of the Cleanse, delve into the Cleanse with a clear intention, and are willing to aim for deep physical, emotional, and lifestyle changes, challenges along the way can feel overwhelming.

That's why before beginning your cleanse it's recommended you get ready by using the simple strategies offered in this chapter. They'll not only help you to ease into the fast-metabolism and detoxing-diet plan, but also support momentum so that you'll stay on track once your cleanse has begun.

Let's make it easy and go step by step.

Step One: Set an Intention

Before beginning any new project, it's important to set an intention. This is especially important when it comes to a lifestyle change. That said, only you know what your specific intention is. Maybe you're on the Metabolism-Boost Cleanse to lose weight, or maybe your goal is to change the way you approach food and/or to eliminate toxins from your life. Maybe you're looking for an overall awareness of what you put in your body and how it functions. Whatever it is, only you can get in touch with the primary purpose of this journey. By setting an intention, you make it clear to yourself and others just what you plan to do. It also redefines what it means to be serious about your dreams. These techniques will help you get there:

Sit quietly for a few minutes and set your intention in your mind's eye. Focus on the benefits you hope to achieve. Repeat them several times. It might also help to write down your goal and then post it in a place where you'll be reminded of your clearest intention.

Share your intention with someone you trust in a way that will supportively hold you accountable for taking action.

Do something today to demonstrate your commitment to your intention. It might be to clean out your pantry of toxic or unhealthy foods, or it might be to simply write down an exercise schedule.

Once you've completed these steps, acknowledge that you did what you said you would and now move on to the next step.

Step Two: Lighten Your Schedule

With a to-do list a mile long, how can you stick to the Metabolism-Boost Cleanse? News flash! You probably can't. That's why it's recommended that you slash any heavy commitments from your schedule not only during your cleanse, but also during the week of preparation. Make a list of what you can release. It helps to be clear about what extra activities and responsibilities you can reschedule and which you absolutely can't postpone. It also benefits you to rally support from friends and family by asking whether you can delegate a few chores. Sweeten the deal by promising you'll have even more energy after the Metabolism-Boost Cleanse so you'll be able to pay back your supporters' favors twofold.

Step Three: Get a Jump on Your Exercise Plan

A crucial component of both kick-starting your metabolism and cleansing is exercise. As described in Chapter Two, certain kinds of exercise are more effective than others, but the choices aren't limiting. If you're not a fan of pumping iron or high-intensity interval training, you can opt for a more subtle approach such as yoga. Let's face it, if you dread an exercise, there's a good chance you'll do everything you can to avoid doing it. That's why it's a good idea to take the time now to commit to a program that suits your sensibility and schedule in a period of 30 minutes daily to devote to it. No excuses.

Studies show exercising in the morning gives your metabolism an extra boost, but if you can't fit it in early in the day, no worries. Just make sure you're done exercising at least four hours before bedtime so your body isn't too hyped up to rest. You want to be able to catch those all-important zzz's.

Step Four: Manage Your Stress

During the preparation week, plus while you're on the Cleanse, it's also a good idea to forgo any big social plans, like dinners out with hard-partying buddies or family get-togethers that you suspect might zap loads of emotional energy. But don't stop there. Be preemptive and commit to practicing some stress-reducing techniques. Of course yoga, meditation, and exercise work wonders, but here are some other simple and enjoyable everyday techniques to consider:

Laugh a little more: Studies show laughing not only makes you feel happier, but also affects your physical body by cooling down the stress response. You don't have to go to a comedy club. Just watching a funny video can do the trick.

Keep a journal: Want to release pent-up emotions? One of the best ways to do it is by writing down how you're feeling. Take note of what's triggering your emotional reaction and what kind of coping tactics you're using to calm down. Don't worry about grammar and spelling. Keep this writing private.

Listen to music: Research points to music's ability to offer mental distraction, lessen muscle tension, and reduce the release of stress hormones.

Look through old photos: Whether they're on your computer or in an album, looking at pictures of happy family gatherings or memorable vacations can actually reduce stress and bring you happiness. Researchers at the United Kingdom's Open University found people's stress levels fell and their moods rose after looking at personal photos.

Think of the good stuff: Every night, review in your mind three things that went well for you that day. They don't have to be earth-shattering events. But allow your mind to revel in the details, and be sure to take note of the role you played in making each happy moment happen. This will help you to realize how much you're actually in charge of your own happiness.

Step Five: Adjust Your Sleep Schedule

It's super important to get a lot of rest during your three days on the Metabolism-Boost Cleanse. Your body will be working hard to jump-start your metabolism while you're detoxing your system, and this process requires lots of rest. The week before your cleanse:

Go to bed the same time every night and set your alarm to awaken at the same time in the mornings, even on weekends.

Make sure you're getting between seven and eight hours of sleep. Take a nap if you need one, but be sure you don't snooze any later in the day than 2 p.m. and for no longer than 30 minutes. Both these factors affect a good night's sleep.

Step Six: Prepare Your Metabolism for Change

It's helpful to ease into as many dietary changes as possible the week before your cleanse. Since it's not helpful to be tempted by foods you won't be eating, give away items in your cupboards and refrigerator you won't need, and replace them with organic whole foods. A shopping list will follow. Meanwhile:

- Eat organic foods as much as possible. Not only vegetables and fruits, but meat, dairy, poultry, and fish.

- Start cutting back on caffeine and alcohol.

- Boost your veggie intake—and not just by eating salads. Include at least three servings a day of lightly steamed broccoli, asparagus, spinach, or similar choices.

⬆ Substitute snacks with fresh juice.

⬆ Replace white rice with brown.

⬆ Cut out processed foods, which include packaged goods, crackers, chips, and salty snacks.

⬆ Nix soy products.

⬆ Cut out carbonated soda—that includes seltzer! Substitute with herbal teas, cold or hot.

⬆ Remove all white sugar and products containing sugar, including cookies, cakes, candy, cereals, and packaged foods.

⬆ Say no to *all* fried foods!

⬆ Greatly reduce or cut out dairy foods. (Although studies show dairy can boost metabolism, it interferes with the effectiveness of cleansing. Hold off on this food group during your cleanse and reintroduce it slowly after the Cleanse.)

- - - - - - - - - - - - -

Be sure to drink at least eight glasses of cold water every day.

- - - - - - - - - - - - -

Step Seven: Feng Shui Your Living Space

Feng shui is an ancient Chinese system of harmonizing human existence with its surrounding environment and is one of the Five Arts of Chinese Metaphysics practices. There are hundreds of principles, but perhaps the most relevant for your cleanse is to create a home that welcomes peace as well as change. Here are some ways to accomplish this goal:

- ⬆ De-clutter: Whether it's your kitchen, living room, bedroom, bathroom, or even the entry way, now is a good time to get rid of anything that isn't visually appealing or essential for living. That includes old newspapers and magazines, as well as dusty knickknacks. Anything worth saving that you don't need or want, donate to charity.

- ⬆ Empty your refrigerator and cupboards of unhealthy and processed foods.

- ⬆ Put your coffee maker away, at least while you're in preparation mode.

- ⬆ Leave plenty of kitchen counter space free for fresh produce.

- ⬆ Clean *everywhere*!

Step Eight: Practice Juicing

If this is a new concept for you, try it out the week before your cleanse. You needn't get an expensive juicer, because the Metabolism-Boost Cleanse concentrates on simple fruit juices rather than vegetable green juices. A standard blender will do the trick. Invite friends or family members to join you in trying out making some of your own favorite fruit juices.

Explore Your Neighborhood: Discover health food stores and farmer's markets.

Step Nine: Go Shopping

You don't want to break the bank preparing for your Metabolism Boost, so don't go overboard. Consider what quantity you'll actually need before filling your sack with goods. Although dried grains and beans can be stored in airtight containers and last for months, you'll only want to buy three days' worth of fresh greens and fruits, as well as proteins like meat and fish. You can replace these foods if the need arises.

SHOPPING LIST

This may not cover everything you'll need for the Metabolism-Boost Cleanse, but it will certainly reduce your need to go on a big shopping trip during the plan. Review Chapter Three for the fast metabolism superfoods and put them on your list. Generally, you'll want to get:

- ⬆ Dried beans/lentils/legumes

- ⬆ Natural sweetener, either stevia, honey, agave, grade-B maple syrup, or brown rice syrup

- ⬆ Herbal teas of your choice

- ⬆ All fresh fruit except bananas; make sure to include lemons

- ⬆ Gluten-free grains, which can include quinoa, brown rice, and buckwheat

- ⬆ Fresh green veggies, including broccoli, spinach, watercress, arugula, kale, etc.

- ⬆ Coconut water

- ⬆ Olive oil

- ⬆ Sea salt

- ↑ Organic eggs (you'll only need the whites)

- ↑ Brown rice milk

- ↑ Ground cinnamon

- ↑ Yellow curry

- ↑ Fresh gingerroot

- ↑ Coconut flakes, unsweetened

- ↑ Steel-cut oats

- ↑ Sprouted-grain bread

- ↑ Grapeseed oil

About 80 percent of the food on shelves of supermarkets today didn't exist 100 years ago.
~ Larry McCleary, author of *Feed Your Brain, Lose Your Belly: A Brain Surgeon Reveals the Weight-Loss Secrets of the Brain-Belly Connection*

Step Ten: Stick to Your Plan

Remember, if you don't prepare properly for the Metabolism-Boost Cleanse, it will be harder to maintain. It will help if you:

Mark it on your calendar: The best time to start your three-day cleanse is on a weekend. Look at your schedule and decide on days that won't interfere with any major upcoming events. I recommend allowing seven to ten days of preparation to ease into the cleanse.

Imagine an obstacle: Let's say the first day you're on the Cleanse you feel exhausted, get a headache, or are tempted to cheat. Now is a good time to figure out coping strategies.

Manage your expectations: Be aware that some people are left particularly vulnerable after their cleanse, so it's not a good idea to end it and then jump right back into your regular routine. Be mindful of how quickly you start adding foods and activities back into your life.

Quiz: How Ready Are You for the Metabolism-Boost Cleanse?

Think you've got it all together and you're primed to start the Cleanse? Well, there may be obvious or hidden factors you might not have dealt with—yet. This quiz can quickly help you identify those issues that might hamper the success of your cleanse and offer tips on how to deal with them now.

1. Which statement most closely reflects my feelings about staying healthy:

   a. For the most part, I think you're dealt a hand and it plays out in your lifetime.

   b. I'm confident that if I devote myself 150 percent to healthy habits, I'll be happier.

   c. I take good care of my mind and body so my life will be deeper and fuller and, hopefully, longer.

2. When it comes to choosing a dish on a menu, the most important thing I consider is:

   a. Flavor.

   b. How many calories are in it.

   c. Whether I think I'll enjoy it during and after.

3. Usually, my "home cooked" meals are:

   a. Either frozen, canned, or take-out.

   b. A big production. I like to try something new almost all the time!

   c. Nothing fancy. Just a simple dish prepared with whatever is fresh and in season.

4. When shopping at the supermarket, I'm more likely to buy whatever:

    a. I'm in the mood for in the moment.

    b. Is on sale, as long as it looks appealing.

    c. Is on my list.

5. About to empty my cupboards of snack foods in preparation for the Cleanse? What's in there?

    a. Chips! Chips! Chips! And salted nuts.

    b. All the ingredients for home-baked cookies, cakes, and pies. Plus store-bought cookies and crackers.

    c. Nuts and dried fruit.

6. Generally, I would describe my level of stress as:

    a. Over the top!

    b. Fluctuates from high to low.

    c. Hums along. I'm often calm.

7. When something goes wrong I tend to:

    a. Eventually forgive the person who is at fault.

    b. Dwell on it forever and blame myself.

c. Try to analyze what part of it was my responsibility and then figure how to prevent it from happening again.

8. My diet success rate is:

a. Not great. I have a tough time sticking to it.

b. Pretty good. But once it's over I tend to gain the weight back—and then some.

c. I don't usually diet.

9. I would say my family:

a. Relies on me for practically everything.

b. Helps out when I ask.

c. Is pretty self-reliant, but when needed we're always there to support each other.

10. Honestly, how often do I exercise?

a. I plan on doing it during the Cleanse, but usually not much.

b. At least once or twice a week.

c. It's just part of my life. I do something at least once a day.

11. I believe that to be thin and healthy, you have to be:

    a. Born lucky.

    b. Be vigilant and on guard 24/7.

    c. Be aware.

12. After I eat something that's "unhealthy," I:

    a. Feel really guilty and figure I've blown it.

    b. Skip food for the rest of the day.

    c. Since it's unusual, I don't make a big deal about it.

13. When it comes to meditation, I:

    a. Think it's probably hocus-pocus, but I'm willing to try it.

    b. Something I've tried, but my mind is always on overdrive.

    c. A practice I use daily or at least frequently.

14. While preparing dinner, I:

    a. Nibble on the ingredients for the meal as I cook.

    b. Plan to eat just what's on my plate, but often end up grabbing seconds.

    c. Hold off eating until I sit down at the table.

15. At a cocktail party I am more likely to:

   a. Sample whatever passes my way and park myself by the bowl of munchies.

   b. Enjoy the hors d'oeuvres but avoid high-fat choices.

   c. Eat only what I consider to be a healthy choice and focus on the conversation.

16. The part of the Cleanse I'm most worried about is being:

   a. Hungry.

   b. Tired.

   c. Overscheduled.

If You Scored Mostly A's: You Need a Self-Esteem Boost

Do you feel like there's someone else in the driver's seat? Are you along just for the ride? Hey, this is *your* life! This is a great opportunity to change your passive approach and gain control of your mental, physical, and emotional well-being. The Metabolism-Boost Cleanse will offer you the tools you need to be in charge. Even though you might hold a deep belief that you can't fight destiny, if you follow the Cleanse, you'll see how much input you really have in your life. Being too passive can prevent you from taking life in the direction you'd like to see it go. Here are some ways to overcome your resistance and boost your self-esteem:

Change your perspective: Do you worry too much about what other people think of you? In the guise of "niceness," you can become a doormat. One way to change this is to stop worrying about what someone else thinks and start paying attention to what you really think.

Focus on what you have going for you: If you're not aware, it can be too easy to undermine your cleanse. You might be telling yourself that you aren't good enough, smart enough, or strong enough. You can end up believing everything is working against you with thoughts like: I was born to be heavy; I can't control my eating; or, I'm addicted to sugar. Sound familiar? Instead, focus on your talents and skills, and ban negative, self-defeating thoughts. When they bubble up, take a deep breath and let them go with your exhale.

Make this your mantra: "I am responsible for my feelings and thoughts." Once you take responsibility for them and accept ownership of them, you have the power to make positive changes in your life.

Try to stay calm: If you're susceptible to emotional highs and lows, you're likely to react impulsively—and that includes eating. For you, de-stressing techniques such as meditation and yoga are especially important.

If You Scored Mostly B's: You Are a Perfectionist

Whatever I accomplish is never really good enough. I feel like a failure unless I give 120 percent. I have a difficult time finishing projects because I think that with more time I could do an even better job. Does this sound like you? Chances are you're a perfectionist. What this means is that rather than working toward improvement, you're trying to be perfect. But that's a trap. Why? Because A) you're human and you'll probably have a slip up or two; and B) you can't possibly do everything that's suggested. You have to make choices based on what's good for you. What makes perfectionism so toxic is that while you're in its grip, you're most focused on avoiding failure. This makes new experiences negative rather than life-changing, affirmative events. What can you do to shoo away this negative attitude and open your heart to unconditional acceptance and in doing so welcome the changes that a successful cleanse will offer you?

Forgive your shortcomings: Nobody is perfect, and everybody has strengths and weaknesses. That's not to say you shouldn't try to change and grow. You can always learn something new or try to improve, but there are times when you'll have to go with what you already know and do what you can based on that. Don't waste time worrying about what you find impossible to do.

Focus on the essentials: Is the real purpose to be perfect or produce a perfect result, or is it to get something done? What really matters? Is it improved health, or are you going to use the Cleanse as a way to prove to yourself that you can "tough it out"?

Let go of other's judgment: Strive for the results that are best for you. Don't let your results be dictated by fear of others' judgment. Accept a broader form of success rather than narrowly defining it to mean you've done everything just right. For example, approach your Metabolism-Boost Cleanse and daily exercise regimen with your eye on health and fitness rather than simply trying to meet a weight loss target.

Reflect on your successes: Think back to something you have done or made that was successful. It may not have been perfect, but it still achieved a goal or objective. Probably you experienced some uncertainty along the way to creating that success. So don't let your reservations and concerns drag you into inaction. Rather than doing a few things perfectly, accomplish many things successfully.

If You Scored Mostly C's: You're in the Zone

You've probably heard the expressions "go with the flow" or "be in the zone." What this means is that you're in a place where it feels so absolutely comfortable, you're able to move with the current and experience bliss while you're doing something. Since you're able to achieve this "zone" state, you won't meet up with roadblocks while on the Metabolism-Boost Cleanse. You have the ability to follow the diet in a "mindless" (no judgment) way, so you'll meet with boundless success. To reinforce your natural flow:

Stay playful: When folks are at play they feel energized. So rather than looking at the Cleanse as a chore or task, think of it as a something fun and challenging, the way you look at other goals in your life.

Strive: Because you take care of yourself, many of the suggestions in the Cleanse are things you've been doing all along. So step it up. Striving for something that challenges your existing skills can lead to an even deeper state of flow. A slight stretching, or attempting something that is a little more advanced than one's current abilities, can also foster a flow state. If you've never done yoga, meditated, or kept a journal, be sure to add at least one of these practices to your cleanse.

Avoid distractions: Since you're someone who likes to multitask and can usually handle lots on your plate with aplomb, you might think you can carry on a heavy schedule while you're cleansing. But that strategy is risky. Studies show distractions can disrupt the flow state. So try to cut back to the essentials. Delegate!

Life is a series of natural and spontaneous changes. Don't resist them—that only creates sorrow. Let reality be reality. Let things flow naturally forward in whatever way they like.

~ Lao Tzu

CHAPTER FIVE

The Metabolism-Boost Cleanse: Three Days to Amazing Grace and Change

The difference between cleansing for a faster metabolism and simply eating for a faster metabolism is it's more of a healthy eating plan than a strict diet. That's because simply eating for a faster metabolism suggests lots of fruits, vegetables, protein, and legumes. It also nixes wheat, corn, dairy, soy, refined sugar, caffeine, alcohol, dried fruit, and fruit juices. So it's got some of the basic cleanse rules down, but with certain differences (such as forbidding fresh fruit juices).

An important rule both programs support? Drinking *plenty* of water. There's an excellent reason for this principle. A research study published in the journal *Obesity* took two groups of overweight adults on a low-calorie diet and gave one group a 17-ounce drink of water before a meal. Over 12 weeks, the group that drank water before the meal lost 44 percent more weight than the control group who did not drink the water.

Remember to drink, drink, drink! Drinking water before a meal helps you to fill up and reduce caloric intake.

So what's different about the Metabolism-Boost Cleanse? *Plenty*. It:

- Takes place over an intensive three-day period.

- Offers specific meal plans.

- Includes fresh fruit juices.

- Incorporates daily activities that are designed to detox you mentally, physically, and emotionally.

- Substantially limits calorie intake, triggering greater weight loss.

🔺 The Metabolism-Boost Cleanse allows your body to focus on repairing itself. After only three days it leaves you:

- Energized
- Upbeat
- Decisive and self-confident
- Thinner
- Calmer and more relaxed
- Physically stronger and more flexible
- With sparkling hair and bright skin

Hopefully, the effects of the Metabolism-Boost Cleanse will help to support the motivation and confidence you need to embark on a permanent change in your lifestyle habits. If followed whole-heartedly, the Cleanse will give you the tools to begin anew and transition to a long-term, healthy way of living.

So what are you waiting for? Let's begin.

What you might need to have handy:

🔺 Journal and a pen

🔺 Meditation cushion or straight-backed chair

🔺 Loofah or natural-fiber body brush

- ⬆ Yoga props, if needed (mat, blocks, etc.)
- ⬆ Sticky notes
- ⬆ Lots of filtered water

Day One

Note: You've already set your circadian rhythm (biological clock) to a regular routine the week before beginning your cleanse, right? Just remember to arise at the same time each morning.

1 Awaken no later than 7 a.m.

2 While still in bed, feel the sheets beneath your body. Gently stretch your arms overhead and your legs down to your toes. Roll slowly from side to side.

3 Try to recall your dreams and write them in your journal. If you can't remember any dreams, record how you're feeling this morning. Look around your room; write about how it looks, such as the light, temperature, view, etc.

4 Get out of bed slowly and consciously.

5 Drink an 8-ounce glass of cold water.

6 Now is a good time to vocalize a life-affirming mantra, such as:

This is the first day of change for the better!

I am going to be healthier and happier!

I have everything I need to live a better life!

Or create any positive affirmation that resonates within you. Say it aloud, then write it on a sticky note and post it where you will see it throughout the day, such as on the refrigerator or your bathroom mirror.

7 Enjoy a cup of Fresh Ginger Tea (page 104).

8 **30 Minutes of Meditation:** Remember, nothing fancy or "heavy." Just sit comfortably with an erect spine on a pillow or a chair that offers straight back support. You can simply watch your breath or recite a simple mantra (like "om") internally. Try not to let your mind get stuck in a particular thought. When one arises, look at it and allow it to float away. Breathe.

9 Sip a glass of cold water.

10 **Shower and Scrub:** Using a loofah or natural-fiber body brush, rub your skin with firm circular strokes before you step into the shower.

Start with your feet and hands, moving up your legs and toward your arms; avoid the delicate areas of your throat and face, as well as any sore spots. Then step into the shower. Finish your shower with a one-minute burst of cold water, which brings the blood circulation to the skin. Doing this daily will support circulation and increase skin detoxification.

11 Enjoy an 8-ounce glass of cold water.

12 **Breakfast:** Choose from one of the following options.

⬆ Oh! Oh! Oatmeal (page 106)

⬆ French Toast Twist (page 107)

13 Enjoy an 8-ounce glass of cold water.

14 While your stomach is fast-metabolizing your breakfast, slow down with a relaxing activity:

Offer a gratitude list.

Read an inspirational book or poems.

Go for a leisurely walk.

Write in your journal.

15 Even if you're not thirsty, sip an 8-ounce glass of cold water.

16 **One Hour of Exercise:** Wait about an hour for your metabolism to work on digesting your breakfast. Now it's time to move your body. As discussed earlier, the type of exercise is your choice. Vigorous exercise increases lymph flow and circulation to help sweat out toxins. For a super-metabolism-boosting workout, opt for HIIT (page 27). Or, for an emphasis on cleansing and detoxifying, choose yoga postures (page 29). The Metabolism-Boost Cleanse is flexible, so if you choose HIIT today, you can opt for yoga tomorrow!

17 Hey, are you drinking enough water? Grab another 8-ounce glass.

18 **Snack:** Choose from one of the following options.

⬆ Blueberry Smoothie (page 105)

⬆ Enjoy a handful of recommended whole raw nuts or seeds, or a mixture.

19 Be sure to enjoy another 8-ounce glass of cold water.

HOW TO CATCH THOSE MIDDAY ZZZ'S

Choose the Right Time: Prime nap time is from 1 p.m. to 2 p.m., when your energy level dips due to a rise in the hormone melatonin at that time of day.

Stay in the Dark: Use a face mask or eye pillow to provide daytime darkness and make your nap more effective.

Not Near Bedtime: Napping within three hours of bedtime may interfere with nighttime sleep.

Shh: Assure that you will not be disturbed for the duration of your nap.

Time It: You will eventually train yourself to nap for the amount of time you set aside. Until then, set an alarm or ask someone to wake you up.

Naps, it should be noted, are not for everyone. Some folks just can't catch a cat nap, and if they do, they wake up groggy and irritable. Insomnia sufferers should also avoid dozing in the afternoon. If this is you, take this time to just rest, recline, and listen to music. Breathe deeply.

20 **Take a Cat Nap:** Napping is actually a normal, healthy behavior, and a natural response to human body rhythms. A short snooze break can dissipate stress and ultimately increase alertness. A recent study in the research journal *Sleep* examined the benefits of naps of various lengths, as well as a schedule with no naps. The results showed that a ten-minute nap produced the most benefit in terms of reduced sleepiness and improved cognitive performance. A nap lasting 30 minutes or longer is more likely to be accompanied by sleep inertia, which is the period of grogginess that sometimes follows sleep.

21 Remember to drink up! Let cold water fill your cup.

22 **Lunch:** Choose from one of the following options.

- Swell Celery Detox Soup (page 108)

- Avocado-Kale Supercleansing Salad (page 108)

23 Enjoy a cup of decaffeinated herbal tea, like chamomile, lemon or raspberry.

24 How about a walk in the sunshine? If there's no sun out, sit near a lamp and envision a bright day.

25 Enjoy an 8-ounce glass of cold water.

Hug yourself: While on your back bend your knees, bring them to your chest, and hug them close to your body with your arms. Hold the pose for 20 to 50 seconds, then release and repeat. This stretch relaxes all the muscles in your body.

26 Time for a Treatment: Chapter Two describes several cleansing and metabolism-boosting treatments, including acupuncture and heat from a sauna or steam room (page 35). You can also opt for a facial (be sure only natural ingredients are used) as well as a "lymphatic drainage" massage.

DO-IT-YOURSELF MASSAGE

Put two tennis balls in a tube sock and place it under your lower back while you're in bed. Position the balls on each side of your spine. Next, with a slow, continuous movement, roll your body back and forth. As the tennis balls knead your muscles, you'll get a deep tissue massage. Drink plenty of water after a massage to help flush toxins.

27 **Snack:** Choose from one of the following.

⬆ Baked Cinnamon Grapefruit (page 105)

⬆ Toasted Coconut (page 106)

— — — — — — — — — — —

Don't forget to thoroughly chew all your meals and snacks. Oh, and drink water!

— — — — — — — — — — —

28 **Get Happy:** The late afternoon is a good time to begin to wind down and enjoy mood-boosting activities. On page 139 you'll find some simple and surprising suggestions to help tickle your funny bone. While you're at it, drink a glass of water.

29 **Eat an Early Dinner:** The later you eat your last meal of the day, the more you will store much of it as fat and thus put on weight. That's because nearer to bedtime, our bodies are pro-grammed to slow down and don't need as much energy. If you eat and go to sleep soon after, food will be stored as fat. In addition, studies show that late-night noshing increases levels of triglycerides, a type of fat found in your blood. When you eat, your body converts any calories it doesn't use right away into triglycerides; high levels may increase your risk of heart attack and

stroke. As if that's not enough, according to the National Institutes of Health, late-night meals can cause indigestion that interferes with sleep. Plus, people who eat late at night tend to eat more. Convinced? While you're on the Metabolism-Boost Cleanse, finish eating by 6 p.m. Here are your menu choices:

- Simple Bowl of Veg and Grain (page 109)
- Grilled Salmon with a Green Side and Quinoa or Brown Rice (page 110)
- Protein stir-fry cooked in olive oil with chicken, green vegetables, and brown rice

30 Enjoy a cup of herbal tea.

31 Write in Your Journal:

Think back to last evening. How different do you feel tonight?

What was a high point of the day?

Did you have any new insights?

Allow yourself to daydream to the max—no holds barred. Now write down your heart-centered fantasy in your journal.

32 Avoid watching TV. Tuck into bed with a good book.

33 Lights out no later than 10 p.m. Sweet dreams!

Day Two

1 Awaken no later than 7 a.m.

2 While still in bed, feel the sheets beneath your body. Gently stretch your arms overhead and your legs down to your toes. Roll slowly from side to side.

3 Try to recall your dreams and write them in your journal. If you can't remember any dreams, record how you're feeling this morning. Look around your room; write about how it looks, such as the light, temperature, view, etc.

4 Get out of bed slowly and consciously.

5 Drink an 8-ounce glass of cold water.

6   Now is a good time to vocalize a life-affirming mantra. Say it aloud, then write it on a sticky note and post it where you will see it throughout the day, such as on the refrigerator or your bathroom mirror.

7   Enjoy a cup of Fresh Ginger Tea (page 104).

8   30 Minutes of Meditation (page 86).

9   Sip a glass of cold water.

10 Shower and Scrub (page 86).

11 Enjoy an 8-ounce glass of cold water.

12 **Breakfast:** Choose from one of the following items.

   ⬆ Oh! Oh! Oatmeal (page 106)

   ⬆ French Toast Twist (page 107)

   ⬆ Spinach Omelet (page 107)

13 Enjoy an 8-ounce glass of cold water.

14 While your stomach is fast-metabolizing your breakfast, slow down with a relaxing activity:

Offer a gratitude list.

Read an inspirational book or poems.

Go for a leisurely walk.

Write in your journal.

15 Even if you're not thirsty, sip some cold water.

16 One Hour of Exercise (page 88).

17 Remember to make sure you're drinking cold water throughout the day!

18 **Snack:** Choose from one of the following items.

- Blueberry Smoothie (page 105)

- Handful of whole raw nuts or seeds, or a mixture of both.

- Sliced apple sprinkled with cinnamon.

19 Enjoy another 8-ounce glass of cold water.

20 Take a Cat Nap (page 90).

21 **Lunch:** Choose from one of the following items.

- ⬆ Swell Celery Detox Soup (page 108)

- ⬆ Avocado-Kale Supercleansing Salad (page 108)

- ⬆ Sweet Quinoa (page 111)

22 Enjoy a cup of herbal tea.

23 How about a walk in the sunshine? If there's no sun out, sit near a lamp and envision a bright day.

24 Enjoy an 8-ounce glass of cold water.

25 Hug Yourself (page 91).

26 Time for a Treatment (page 91).

27 Reflect on your cleanse experience thus far and be happy with all the good you're doing for your body and mind by ridding your body of toxins and nourishing yourself with delicious whole foods.

28 **Eat an Early No-Fuss Dinner:** Choose from one of the following options.

- ⬆ Simple Bowl of Veg and Grain (page 109)

- ⬆ Grilled Salmon (page 110)

- ⬆ Protein-stir fry made with lean protein such as chicken, green vegetables, and brown rice

29 Enjoy a cup of herbal tea.

30 Write in Your Journal:

Think back to last evening. How different do you feel tonight?

What was a high point of the day?

Did you have any new insights?

Allow yourself to daydream to the max—no holds barred. Now write down your heart-centered fantasy in your journal.

31 Avoid watching TV. Tuck into bed with a good book.

32 Lights out no later than 10 p.m.

Day Three

1 Awaken no later than 7 a.m.

2 While still in bed, feel the sheets beneath your body. Gently stretch your arms overhead and your legs down to your toes. Roll slowly from side to side.

3 Try to recall your dreams and write them in your journal. If you can't remember any dreams, record how you're feeling this morning. Look around your room; write about how it looks, such as the light, temperature, view, etc.

4 Get out of bed slowly and consciously.

5 Drink an 8-ounce glass of cold water.

6 Now is a good time to vocalize a life-affirming mantra. Say it aloud, then write it on a sticky note and post it where you will see it throughout the day, such as on the refrigerator or your bathroom mirror.

7 Enjoy a cup of Fresh Ginger Tea (page 104).

8 30 Minutes of Meditation (page 86).

9 Sip a glass of cold water.

10 Shower and Scrub (page 86).

11 Enjoy an 8-ounce glass of cold water.

12 **Breakfast:** Choose from one of the following options.

⬆ Oh! Oh! Oatmeal (page 106)

⬆ French Toast Twist (page 107)

⬆ Spinach Omelet (page 107)

13 Enjoy an 8-ounce glass of cold water.

14 While your stomach is fast-metabolizing your breakfast, slow down with one of these relaxing activities:

Offer a gratitude list.

Read an inspirational book or poems.

Go for a leisurely walk.

Write in your journal.

15 Even if you're not thirsty, sip some cold water.

16 One Hour of Exercise (page 88).

17 Are you remembering to drink enough water? Sip another cold glassful.

18 **Snack:** Choose from one of the following options.

- Blueberry Smoothie (page 105)

- Handful of whole raw nuts or seeds, or a mixture of both

- Sliced apple sprinkled with cinnamon

19 Enjoy another 8-ounce glass of cold water.

20 Take a Cat Nap (page 90).

21 **Lunch:** Choose from one of the following options.

- Swell Celery Detox Soup (page 108)

- Avocado-Kale Supercleansing Salad (page 108)

- Sweet Quinoa (page 111)

22 Enjoy a cup of herbal tea.

23 How about a walk in the sunshine? If there's no sun out, sit near a lamp and envision a bright day.

24 Drink another glass of cold water.

25 Hug Yourself (page 91).

26 Time for a Treatment (page 91).

27 Be happy. "Happiness" mood neurotransmitters in your brain affect how well you'll stick to a cleanse. If you're happy you're more likely to eat better and exercise. Conversely, high stress levels cause your body to release the hormone cortisol which makes us crave unhealthy comfort foods like pizza, cupcakes and ice cream.

28 **Eat an Early No-Fuss Dinner:** Choose from one of the following options.

- Simple Bowl of Veg and Grain (page 109)

- Grilled Salmon with a Green Side and Quinoa or Brown Rice (page 110)

- Protein-stir fry made with lean protein such as chicken, green vegetables, and brown rice

29 Enjoy a cup of herbal tea.

30 Write in Your Journal:

> *Think back to last evening. How different do you feel tonight?*
>
> *What was a high point of the day?*
>
> *Did you have any new insights?*

Allow yourself to daydream to the max—no holds barred. Now write down your heart-centered fantasy in your journal.

31 Avoid watching TV. Tuck into bed with a good book.

32 Lights out no later than 10 p.m.

We must walk consciously only part way toward our goal, and then leap in the dark to our success.

~ Henry David Thoreau

CHAPTER SIX

Metabolism-Boost Recipes

If you're ready to embark on the journey toward cleansing your life and boosting your metabolism, here you'll find all the recipes you'll need for success.

Cleanse Recipes

The following dishes are everything you'll need during your three-day Metabolism-Boost Cleanse.

DRINKS

Fresh Ginger Tea
Serves 2

4 to 6 thin slices peeled raw gingerroot
1½ to 2 cups water
Juice of ½ lime, or to taste (optional)
Up to 2 teaspoons grade B maple syrup,
   to taste

Remember that the thinner you slice the ginger, the more flavorful your tea will be. Boil the ginger in the water for at least 10 minutes. Remove from the heat and add the lime juice, if using, and maple syrup to taste.

Blueberry Smoothie
Serves 1

> 1 cup fresh blueberries
> ½ cup unsweetened brown rice milk
> 3 ice cubes

Combine the blueberries, rice milk, and ice cubes in a blender and blend until smooth. Drink immediately.

SNACKS

Baked Cinnamon Grapefruit
Serves 2

> 1 pink grapefruit
> ¼ teaspoon ground cinnamon

Preheat the oven to 375°F. Peel and section the grapefruit. Sprinkle with the cinnamon. Bake for 20 minutes, until the grapefruit has caramelized.

Toasted Coconut
Serves 3 to 4

> 2 cups of unsweetened raw coconut
> flakes

Preheat oven to 325°F. Spread coconut flakes on a baking sheet in a thin layer and bake in preheated oven. Bake for no more than eight minutes. Check after five minutes as they may brown faster.

BREAKFASTS

Oh! Oh! Oatmeal
Serves 1

> ½ cup steel-cut oats
> ½ cup unsweetened brown rice milk
> ½ teaspoon ground cinnamon
> ½ cup fresh blueberries

In a small saucepan over medium-high heat, combine the oats, rice milk, and cinnamon. Bring water to a boil in a saucepan and stir in your oats. Reduce heat to a simmer and cook oats until soft, 20 to 30 minutes, stirring occasionally. Scoop into your favorite bowl and top with blueberries.

French Toast Twist
Serves 1

    1 tablespoon grapeseed oil
    1 egg white
    ¼ teaspoon ground cinnamon
    1 slice whole-grain sprouted bread
    Drizzle of maple syrup

Heat the grapeseed oil in a medium skillet over medium-high. Whisk together the egg and cinnamon in a wide, shallow bowl. Place the bread into the mixture and be sure both sides are fully coated. Cook until brown on both sides. Serve with drizzle of maple syrup. Chew thoroughly and consciously.

Spinach Omelet
Serves 1

    ¼ teaspoon extra-virgin olive oil
    1 egg
    1 cup steamed spinach

Heat the olive oil in a small skillet over medium heat. Quickly whisk the egg in a small bowl and pour into the skillet. When the edges firm, lay the steamed spinach on top, fold the egg in half over the spinach, and remove from the heat.

SALADS

Avocado-Kale Supercleansing Salad
Serves 2

½ head kale, torn into 2-inch pieces
½ cup arugula
1 tablespoon fresh lemon juice
1 avocado, diced
1 teaspoon chia seeds
Dash of cayenne pepper
Salt, to taste

Toss the kale, arugula, and avocado in a large bowl with your hands, squeezing to coat the kale leaves with the avocado. Add the remaining ingredients, toss again, and serve.

SOUPS

Swell Celery Detox Soup
Serves 4

4 chopped celery stalks
3 handfuls fresh chopped spinach
1 medium chopped Vidalia onion

2 garlic cloves
½ teaspoon ground ginger
½ teaspoon ground cumin
1 teaspoon dried mint
1½ cup water
½ cup of coconut milk
Salt and pepper to taste

Boil water in a pot and add sea salt to your taste. Add chopped celery, spinach, onion, ginger, cumin, and mint to the pot. Cook over medium heat, covered with a lid, for 15 minutes until they soften. Turn off the heat, add 2 whole garlic cloves. Blend until pureed. Pour the soup into the plates, drizzle with coconut milk. Sprinkle with freshly ground black pepper.

ENTRÉES

Simple Bowl of Veg and Grain
Serves 4

3 cups lightly steamed broccoli
½ to 1 cup cooked quinoa
½ cup cooked lentils

Mix together and enjoy!

Grilled Salmon
serves 2

> 1lb fresh salmon
> 2 tablespoons olive oil
> salt and pepper, to taste
> garlic, to taste

Rub olive oil onto the salmon. Grill the first side for 5 minutes, flip and grill the reverse side for 3 minutes. Serve with a side of steamed greens, such as spinach, kale, or broccoli, and quinoa or brown rice.

Grilled Salmon with a Green Side and Quinoa or Brown Rice
Serves 6

> 1½ salmon fillets
> ½ squeezed lemon
> Pinch salt and pepper
> Garlic powder to taste
> ¼ cup olive oil

Season fillets to taste with lemon, garlic and salt and pepper. Preheat grill for medium heat. Lightly spread the olive oil on the grill. Place the fillets on the grill and cook for 6 to 8 minutes on each side.

Side of greens can be salad, or steamed broccoli.

Sweet Quinoa

Serves 1

> ¼ cup uncooked quinoa
> ½ teaspoon grade B maple syrup
> ¼ cup chopped almonds
> Juice of ½ orange
> ½ teaspoon freshly grated orange zest

Cook the quinoa according to the package instructions. Remove from the heat and immediately transfer to a large bowl. Add the maple syrup and toss to combine. Cover and set aside for 5 minutes to allow the syrup to soak in. Add the remaining ingredients to the bowl and toss to combine.

More on Your Metabolism-Boost Menu

You've followed the Metabolism-Boost Cleanse for three days. Now allow yourself to imagine the potential of continuing forever on your path of well-being. If you're thinking, "Whoa, that's not so easy!" you're right. For most of us living in today's junk food culture, staying committed to healthy habits takes focused commitment. And it's unreasonable to expect any busy individual with family, relationship, and career commitments to devote a tremendous amount of time to any special dietary program. Three days is one thing, a lifetime is another.

The good news is that you can blend beneficial food basics into your daily life in simple ways and continue to reap the benefits of a fast-metabolism, non-toxic diet. You can continue to make healthy lifestyle choices without making a huge deal about it.

Let's quickly review the basic food rules for a fast, clean metabolism:

- ⬆ Never skip breakfast.

- ⬆ Drink plenty of water. Definitely a glass before meals. Make it cold for an optimal metabolism boost.

- ⬆ Enjoy at least two snacks daily.

- ⬆ Nix refined sugar.

- ⬆ Ban, or at least, limit processed foods.

- ⬆ Opt whenever you can for organic fruits, vegetables, and proteins.

- ⬆ Stop eating early in the evening when possible.

⬆ Chew each bite at least 20 times.

⬆ Make one meal a day a Metabolism-Boost Cleanse dish.

That's not so difficult, right?

I was eating bad stuff. Lots of sugar and carbs, junk food all the time. It makes you very irritated.
~ Avril Lavigne

Eating for Health: Twenty Delicious Recipes

The best plan is the easiest one. Rather than think you have to adhere to a strict diet every time you put something in your mouth, relax. As long as you stick with the basic rules listed above, you'll be doing your metabolism and the rest of your body a big favor. One Metabolism-Boost Cleanse dish a day does the trick. Even better news? It can be an entrée, juice, soup, or snack—even a dessert.

In this chapter you'll find simple recipes for every meal of the day. Read them through, and when something makes your mouth water, that's the dish to try first. Bon appétit!

DRINKS

Green Giant Juice
Serves 2 glasses

Handful of kale (or any other dark, leafy
green)
Handful of any other dark, leafy green
Rib of celery
½ medium peeled cucumber
Small handful of cilantro
1 inch fresh gingerroot, chopped
Pinch of sea salt
Juice of ½ lemon
1 cup coconut water
⅛ teaspoon maple syrup
2 ice cubes, crushed

Add ingredients together in a blender until smooth
and creamy.

Three-Ingredient Juice
Serves 1 glass

2 Baldwin or Burgundy apples, cored
1 lime, peeled
4 carrots, peeled

Add ingredients together in a juicer until juiced to
perfection.

DON'T DETOX AS A PURGE

If you overindulge on a long weekend or vacation, don't look to a detox or cleanse to erase those calories. Emotionally using cleanses and detoxes this way can become a lot like other methods of purging, including overexercise, or taking laxatives or diuretics—it can feel like something you don't want to do, and know isn't healthy, but feel like you have to do in order to undo the effects of overeating.

Apple-Spinach Elixir
Serves 2 glasses

2 apples, cored
1 orange, peeled
3 cups spinach
1 medium peeled cucumber

Cut all the ingredients as needed. Puree it all in a blender and enjoy.

SNACKS

Avocado Avalanche
Serves 2

> 1 avocado
> 1 teaspoon tamari

Cut the avocado in half and take out the pit. Score both halves and drizzle the tarmari over them.

Four Fruit Kebabs with Chocolate
Serves 2

> 1 apple
> 2 mandarins, peeled
> 3 slices pineapple
> ½ (½-ounce) dark chocolate bar, melted

Slice all the fruit into bite-size pieces and stick on two kebab skewers. Then drizzle with the chocolate. Eat it right away or let it sit at room temperature until the chocolate hardens.

Apple Sandwich
Serves 1

  1 apple
  1 teaspoon unsalted almond butter

Thinly slice the apple from top to bottom and core each piece. Then layer each slice with nut butter and stack together.

Chia Pudding
Serves 1

  2 tablespoons chia seeds
  ½ cup water
  1 tablespoon hemp seeds
  1 tablespoon ground flaxseed
  ½ teaspoon ground cinnamon
  ½ teaspoon vanilla extract
  ¼ teaspoon maple syrup

In a small bowl, stir together the chia seeds and water. Let it sit for a few minutes to gelatinize, then add the other ingredients.

SALADS

Gorgeous Green Salad
Serves 5 to 6

¼ medium peeled cucumber
¼ medium red onion
5 cups or more fresh salad greens
1 handful fresh herbs like basil, cilantro,
   lemon balm, or rosemary, or a mixture
1 avocado, pitted and sliced
Juice of ½ lemon
Sea salt

Chop the cucumber, onion, and herbs, and mix with
the greens. Drop in chunky slices of avocado. Drizzle
with lemon juice and toss. Season with salt to taste.

Crunchy Cabbage Salad
Serves 2

½ small green cabbage, finely shredded
1 cup snow peas, chopped
1 bunch green onions, chopped
½ cup sunflower seeds, lightly toasted for
   added crunch, if desired
½ cup of flaked almonds, lightly toasted
   for added crunch, if desired
½ cup cilantro, chopped (optional)
Juice of ½ lemon

Place all the ingredients in a large bowl, and drizzle
with the fresh lemon juice. Toss to combine.

CAN I DO THE CLEANSE GLUTEN-FREE?

It's actually really easy to do the Metabolism-Boost Cleanse gluten-free. There's no wheat on the diet already, and there are plenty of other gluten-free grains to choose from, like quinoa, buckwheat, brown rice, or even wild rice. It may be difficult for you to find a sprouted grain bread that will work (that doesn't contain sugar, soy, or corn), but you can choose another grain.

Garlic-Chickpea Extravaganza
Serves 4

Salad:
5 cucumber slices, peeled
½ cup chickpeas
4 to 5 cups kale, in bite-size pieces, destemmed

Dressing:
1 tablespoon French mustard
1 tablespoon tamari
3 tablespoons water
½ clove garlic
1 tablespoon miso
1 tablespoon maple syrup

To make the salad, toss all the ingredients together in a large bowl. Add all the dressing ingredients together and blend until smooth. Pour the dressing over the greens and toss to combine.

SOUPS

Coconut Curry Squash Soup
Serves 8

> 5 cups peeled, cubed raw butternut squash
> 2 cups coconut milk
> 1 orange, peeled
> ½ yellow onion, coarsely chopped
> Drizzle of maple syrup, to sweeten
> 1 tablespoon yellow curry powder
> 3 thin (1-inch) slices peeled ginger
> 1 clove garlic
> 1 teaspoon ground cinnamon
> ½ cup vegetable stock
> Water, as needed

Blend all ingredients together in blender until smooth, adding water as needed for consistency. Store any leftovers in an airtight container in the freezer.

Corn, Garlic, and Tomato Soup
Serves 2 or 3

> 1 tomato
> ⅓ cup sweet corn kernels, fresh or frozen
> 1 to 3 cloves garlic
> Handful of chopped walnuts
> Teaspoon of chia seeds
> 1½ cups hot water
> ½ to 1 avocado, chopped
> Salt
> Fresh or dried dill, for garnish

Blend the tomato, corn, garlic, walnuts, chia seeds, water, and half of whatever amount of avocado you're using until smooth. Pour into a serving bowl. Add salt to taste, and top with remaining chopped avocado and dill.

ENTRÉES

Homemade "Sushi"
Serves 2

> 1 bell pepper
> 1 rib celery
> ½ avocado
> ¼ cup tahini sauce or peanut butter

3 big leaves cooked greens (spinach, kale,
etc.) or nori sheets
1 cup sprouts

Cut all the bell pepper, celery, and avocado into
matchsticks. Spread the tahini or peanut butter
onto the inside of each leaf of greens. Spread the
sprouts all over the leaf, followed by the veg sticks
and avocado on one side. Put a bit more sauce on
the opposite side and roll up. Then cut the roll into
sushi-sized pieces.

Zucchini Noodles
Serves 2

Noodles:
2 small zucchinis

Sauce:
¼ cup raw pumpkin seeds
1 to 2 cloves garlic, chopped
¼ cup basil leaves or other fresh herbs
2 tablespoons dates, chopped
Water, as needed

To make the noodles, slice the zucchinis with a
spiral slicer and set aside in a large bowl. To make
the sauce, add all the ingredients together and blend
until smooth, adding water to thin as needed. Evenly
coat the noodles with the sauce. Let marinate 5 five
minutes and then enjoy.

Kale Pesto & Yam Tofu
Serves 2

Kale Pesto:
5 cups kale, torn into bite-size pieces
½ cup pine nuts
1 tablespoon walnut oil
Salt, to taste
Water, as needed

Baked Yam and Tofu:
1 medium yam, peeled
1 (12-ounce) package soft tofu
1 tablespoon extra-virgin olive oil
1 teaspoon grade B maple syrup
Salt

To make the kale pesto, place all the ingredients in a blender and puree, adding water as needed for consistency. To make the baked yam and tofu, preheat the oven to 350°F. Cut the yam and tofu into bite-size chunks and toss in the olive oil, maple syrup, and salt to taste. Bake for 20 to 30 minutes, until the yam is soft. Serve with the kale pesto.

Curried Lentils with Onions
Serves 6

1 cup French lentils or black lentils
3½ cups water, divided
4 tablespoon coconut oil
2 teaspoons yellow curry powder

2 medium sweet yellow onions (Vidalia),
   thinly sliced (about 3 cups)
3 tablespoons cilantro leaves, loosely
   packed

Place lentils and 3 cups of the water in a small pot.
Cover and bring to a boil over medium heat. Reduce
to a simmer and cook, covered, for about 30 minutes.
In a large pan, heat the oil over medium and add the
curry and onions. Sauté until the onions are golden
brown. Add the remaining ½ cup water and cook for
another 10 minutes. When the lentils are done, combine with the onions in the pan and mix well. Toss in
the cilantro and season with salt to taste.

STRESS-FIGHTING FOODS

Roasted Salmon with Mustard and Dill
Serves 1

1 salmon fillet (about 6 ounces)
½ lemon, or to taste
Extra-virgin olive oil, for drizzling
Salt and black pepper, to taste
⅛ teaspoon garlic powder
½ tablespoon stone-ground mustard
2 teaspoons fresh dill

Preheat the oven to 375°F and lightly oil a roasting
pan. Squeeze the juice of ½ lemon over the salmon

fillet. Drizzle with the olive oil. Sprinkle with salt, pepper, and garlic powder. Spread the mustard evenly over the top of the salmon, and sprinkle the dill over the mustard, coating the salmon generously. Place the salmon skin-side down on the prepared pan and roast in the oven until the salmon is fork-tender and flakes easily, about 10 minutes, depending on thickness.

Simple Roast Chicken
Serves 4

> 4 bone-in, skin-on chicken breasts
> Salt and pepper, to taste
> ¼ teaspoon dried oregano
> Sprinkle of garlic powder
> Paprika, to taste
> 1 parsnip, peeled and sliced
> 1 carrot, peeled and sliced
> 1 sweet potato, peeled and sliced
> ½ butternut squash, peeled and sliced
> 1 red onion, peeled and cut into wedges
> 3 cloves garlic, sliced
> Extra-virgin olive oil, for drizzling

Preheat the oven to 375°F. Season the chicken with salt, pepper, oregano, garlic powder, and paprika and place in an ovenproof roasting dish. Arrange the parsnip, carrot, sweet potato, ½ butternut squash, and onion around the chicken. Throw in the garlic, and drizzle the vegetables with a little olive oil. Roast until the chicken is cooked through, about 40 minutes.

STRESS-FIGHTING FOODS

When we substitute our unhealthy cravings for smart choices, we can calm our nerves and stay cool as a cucumber. To reduce stress and anxiety, try these power foods:

Nuts: Research shows a connection between selenium deficiency and increased anxiety, depression, and fatigue. You can turn it around by eating nuts (particularly Brazil nuts). Just a handful a day does the trick. Other sources of selenium include shitake mushrooms, tuna, cod, and salmon.

Spinach: Popeye's snack of choice contains heaps of magnesium, which helps to keep your nerves steady and your muscles in a relaxed state. Your body will let you know if you don't have enough magnesium, not only by pumping up your anxiety, but with muscle tension, cramps, and fatigue. Try to include 1 cup of fresh spinach or ½ cup of cooked spinach to your diet each day.

Dark chocolate: The amino acid tryptophan is essential in helping the body to create serotonin, a neurochemical that eases anxiety. Lucky us—dark chocolate is rich in tryptophan! Other foods that contain tryptophan include almonds, sunflower seeds, sesame seeds, nuts, legumes, dark turkey meat, and red meat.

Herbs: Opt for basil, which is an excellent source of magnesium and helps muscles and blood vessels to relax. As a bonus, it also contains antibacterial and anti-inflammatory properties that are useful if you have rheumatoid arthritis or inflammatory bowel conditions. Other calming herbs include lemon balm and chamomile, both of which you can drink in a tea.

Oats: Complex carbohydrates enhance the absorption of tryptophan, which is in turn used to manufacture serotonin. To get the soothing effect from oats, eat them together with some proteins, such as nuts or seeds.

Broccoli: Rich in potassium and beta-carotene, as well as the vitamins C and E, broccoli not only gives your immune system a boost, but it's the perfect food to relax your nerves. Other sources of potassium include avocado, banana, kale, brussels sprouts, cabbage, winter squash, eggplant, and tomatoes.

DESSERTS

Peanut Butter Cups
Makes 5 peanut butter cups

   4 ounces dark chocolate
   2 teaspoons nutritional yeast
   ⅓ cup peanut butter, smooth and
      unsalted

Melt the chocolate in a double boiler. Meanwhile, mix the nutritional yeast with the peanut butter until smooth. Pour a dot of melted chocolate into the bottom of each of 5 silicone cupcake molds (you should have used nearly half the chocolate when finished with this step). Put almost a tablespoon of peanut butter in each mold, but don't let it touch the sides. Next, pour the rest of the chocolate among the molds. Be sure it covers all the peanut butter and the sides. Refrigerate for a couple of hours, until hardened, then take them out of their molds.

Coconut Lemon Bars
Makes about 12 bars

   Base:
   ¾ cup oats (or buckwheat groats, to
      make it gluten-free)
   ¾ cup shredded coconut, unsweetened
   ¾ cup whole dates, pitted

Lemon Layer:
⅓ cup melted coconut oil
¼ cup grade B maple syrup
Juice of 3 lemons
½ cup shredded coconut
1 or 2 bananas
Finely ground unsweetened coconut
    flakes, for garnish

To make the base, pulse the oats or buckwheat groats and shredded coconut together in a food processor until it turns into coarse flour. Add the dates and process until it all sticks together. Press into the bottom of a square baking pan and put in the fridge.

To make the lemon layer, add all the ingredients together and blend until smooth. Spread evenly on to the base and refrigerate overnight. The next day, cut into squares and sprinkle with finely ground coconut flakes for a powdered sugar effect.

Eating for Metabolism When You're Dining Out

Home cooking not only helps us keep our diet in check, but it's also a way to be creative and productive. It makes us happy. But what about when we can't be at home to cook? No problem. Going out for meals is a terrific way to socialize. And if you're lucky there will be weddings, birthday celebrations, business meetings, and get-togethers with friends and romantic partners. Are you worried that eating out will sabotage your new approach to eating? Don't be.

With a little bit of strategizing, as well as keeping your eating basics in mind, you'll be able to enjoy eating out while still adhering to your new approach to food.

Here are a few tips:

- ⬆ If you know where you're going to be eating, check out the restaurant's menu online beforehand. It's less pressure to scope out the choices at home than with a waiter breathing down your neck. Match up meals with the foods on the Metabolism-Boost Cleanse to decide in advance which comes closest.

- ⬆ Decide what to order before you sit down. By setting your mind on the best choice before you get to the restaurant, you avoid making last-minute mistakes.

- ⬆ If the restaurant that's been chosen has very few options for you, do a Web search to find nearby alternatives and suggest it to your companions.

- ⬆ If you're staying in a hotel, check out the nearby restaurant choices online. You can also call ahead and have your room's mini bar cleaned out so there won't be any temptation.

WHAT IF IT'S CATERED?

If you're at a wedding or business meeting, you can count on it being catered with limited food choices. The menu has already been planned. But you can still make good choices.

- ⬆ Call the caterer. In hotels and resorts, the staff is used to accommodating people with differing dietary needs or allergies. Call the catering department several days in advance and inquire about the menu. Explain that you have some dietary restrictions and ask how they can work with you. Most will be happy to provide veggies and meats without butter or oil, as well as wheat-free options. If they agree to make you a special meal, call to confirm the day before the event. Sharing the reasons why you're asking for these changes can help get them invested in helping you.

- ⬆ For events with buffets, scope out the whole buffet first without picking up a plate. Decide on the best options. Then make your way through the line.

- Ask for fresh lemon instead of the planned salad dressing.

- Bring along your own snacks so you won't be tempted to go crazy at the dessert table.

BE POLITE, BUT DON'T BE AFRAID TO ASK QUESTIONS!

Wait staff is there to not only take orders, but to answer questions. Don't be shy!

- Explain to the waiter that you have some dietary restrictions and ask for his or her help.

- Ask how menu items are prepared. Can they be made without sauces/butter/oil?

- Ask for veggies on the side instead of potatoes.

- Skip the bread basket. Ask the waiter to take it away, or at least keep it at the end of the table. Or better yet, do not have the waiter bring it in the first place.

I had these recipes that say do this, do that. Who makes these rules?

~ Emeril Lagasse

CHAPTER SEVEN

Eleven Power Tips for Staying Healthy in the Fast Lane

In my dreams, I'm spending a week unwinding at a five-star spa. In reality, if I don't focus on what's most important, I'm lucky if I find the time to pamper myself with hand cream. This kind of lifestyle is exciting on many levels, but it can really do a number on your health and well-being. Not only can it interfere with your commitment to keep your diet metabolically fast and nontoxic, but it can sabotage your life, unhinging your emotional, spiritual, and psychic balance.

In this final chapter, a spotlight shines on those elements in your life that might cast shadows on your brightest hopes. You'll be able to identify your personal bugaboos with two simple quizzes and get personalized tips on ways to combat the obstacles that stand in the way of your inner and outer makeover. None of the suggestions is impossible to implement in your life. For example, you needn't schedule long retreat time to reap the benefits of deep relaxation and rejuvenation.

First things first. Here are the eleven powerful steps you can take to move in a positive direction.

Step One: Take It Slow

Studies show that taking it slow is good for your health and well-being. It lowers inflammation, stabilizes blood pressure, keeps glucose levels steady, helps in decision making, and ultimately makes you happier. So, how can we put the brakes on a natural tendency to be impatient?

Give It a Day: Take an entire day when you make it your goal to be patient. At the end of it, write down all the ways it helped you. Like any skill, developing patience takes practice. Try it once a week, until you can build up a tolerance for taking it easy.

Breathe: When you're frustrated and in a hurry, stop. Take several deep breaths. For example, if you're in a long line at the grocery store or in heavy traffic, make the decision to pause and not get worked up.

Remind yourself that getting impatient won't make things move along any faster, so why get stressed for nothing? Now breathe deeply.

Practice Thinking before Speaking: When we're hurrying or letting emotions run wild, we often blurt out the first thought that comes into our heads. Next time, hold your tongue, consider what you want to say first, and think about the consequences. You can avoid hurting or offending others by slowing down reaction time.

Expect the Unexpected: Yes, you have plans, but things don't always work out as planned. Accept the twists and turns in life gracefully. Keep your expectations realistic. This applies not only to circumstances, but also the behavior of those around you.

Step Two: Gain the Power to Say No

You may be feeling overwhelmed with family responsibilities, health problems, work issues, household chores—and then someone asks you to do a favor. Your inner voice is screaming, "No! No! No!" But what do you answer instead? "Yes." Sound familiar? Taking on more than you can, or really *want* to handle, can cause unhealthy stress. Learn to say "No!" Here's how to do it:

Set Priorities: Take a look at your current obligations and overall responsibilities. Ask yourself: Is this new commitment really important to me? If it's something you feel strongly about, by all means do it. If not, take a pass.

Weigh the Stress that Comes with Yes: Is this a long– or short-term commitment? For example, making a batch of cookies for the community center's bake sale will take far less time than heading up the fundraising committee. Don't say yes if it will mean months of added stress. Instead, look for other ways to pitch in.

Kiss Guilt Good-bye: Don't agree to a request because of feelings of guilt or obligation. Remind yourself that going this route is a surefire way to add stress and resentment to your life.

Sleep on It: No matter what you're asked to do, before you give your answer, take a day to think about the request and how it fits in with your current commitments.

Just Say No!: It's powerful, but don't shy away from this two-letter word. If you use substitute phrases, such as, "I'm not sure" or "I don't think I can," they can be interpreted to mean that you might say yes later. You'll just prolong the agony.

Make It Short: State your reason for refusing the request, but don't go on about it. Avoid elaborate justifications or explanations.

Tell the Truth: Don't fabricate reasons to get out of an obligation. The truth is always the best way to turn down a friend or family member. Chances are they will understand completely.

Step Three: Feel Gratitude

It's tough when struggling with a crisis to feel gratitude, but several studies have shown that good feelings such as having a new appreciation for life or seeing the upsides to a healthier lifestyle will not only help us deal with our problems, but also help to boost our health. Consider this: Researchers at the University of Connecticut found that patients who saw benefits and gains from their heart attack experienced a lower risk of having another one. Here are five simple ways you can develop an attitude of gratitude:

Note All the Good Things in Your Life: Even small events matter. For practice, keep a "good things" journal and write down all the wonderful things that happen to you during the day, from a child offering a smile to the sun shining. During times when it feels impossible to conjure up feelings of gratitude, open your journal and read through it for inspiration.

Spend Time with Positive People: Optimism and feelings of gratitude are contagious. Likewise, if you surround yourself with negative people who are always complaining, it will be difficult for you to stay in an upbeat mood.

Be Generous: By giving to others, especially with your time, your mind will focus on what you have rather than what you don't. Unfortunately, most people focus on receiving, which only makes their mind focus on what they lack. Research also shows that people who volunteer are generally happier—and live longer.

Write to Someone Who Really Matters: Dr. Martin Seligman of the University of Pennsylvania recommends writing a 300-word letter to someone who changed your life for the better. Be specific about what the person did and how it affected you.

Be Clear: Don't confuse gratitude with indebtedness. Sure, you may feel obliged to return a favor, but that's not gratitude, at least not the way psychologists define it. Indebtedness is more of a negative feeling and doesn't yield the same benefits as gratitude, which inclines you to be nice to anyone, not just a benefactor.

Step Four: Boost Your Emotional Resiliency

We all suffer from stress at one point or another, but managing it can make a huge improvement in your life. There are four ways to instantly put a lid on high anxiety:

Visualization: Imagine watching the sunset, sitting on a beach, or floating on a lake, and reap the same stress-releasing rewards as if you were actually lolling on the beach. Studies show when you imagine paradise, the natural brain tranquilizer serotonin is released, lowering blood pressure and heart rate.

Shoot the Breeze: Talking about your problems can help sort through what's really eating at you. Make sure your confidante is a sound listener who doesn't interrupt and can be trusted to offer solid advice.

LOL: Watch a funny movie or read a humorous book. Lots of scientific studies prove when you laugh out loud, the anti-stress hormone, dopamine, is pumped through the body. Belly laughing detoxes your lungs, offering the same beneficial effects of deep breathing!

Cool Off: Open a window, stand by the fan or air conditioner, or splash cool water on your face. Lowering your body temperature is a proven method for slowing heart rate and clearing your mind.

If you're feeling overwhelmed, ask for a hug! A University of North Carolina study confirms hugs boost the stress-fighting hormone oxytocin.

Step Five: Relieve Stress Big Time

Muscle tension, headaches and tummy problems are the most common symptoms of stress, but you can banish them with these power tips:

Unwind With Progressive Muscle Relaxation (PMR): Sit or lie down comfortably, then tense and relax one part of your body at a time. Start with your fingers and end with your toes, but don't forget your eyes and mouth. Studies show when you learn how your muscles feel when tensed, you're better able to learn how to focus and relax them.

Come to Your Senses: Surround yourself with calming and energizing scents like lavender, rose, jasmine, eucalyptus, and sage.

Tune In: Lift your spirits and unload your worries by listening to gospel, choral, or classical tunes. The calming effect of music is so powerful that dentists use it during drilling. Research proves music also accelerates the body's production of the feel-good brain chemical, endorphin.

Gazing at fish swimming in a tank lowers blood pressure!

Step Six: Simply Sip Tea

Did you know there's another natural treatment that can soothe your nerves, and you don't have to get off your comfy couch to reap its benefits? What's this secret stress-buster? It's in a cup of herbal tea.

You'll find various combinations of these herbs as calming teas in your grocery store or in pill form in your local health food store. But keep in mind, herbal teas can be powerful. Make sure to check with your doctor if you're taking medications to clear them for possible dangerous interactions. That said, here are the top stress-reducing teas:

Chamomile: Dried chamomile flowers have been used throughout the ages: The ancient Egyptians worshipped them, and the ancient Greeks actually considered them sacred. A sedative, relaxant, and anti-depressant, this soothing herb is also used to relieve insomnia and nervous indigestion, because it contains essential volatile oils and flavonoids, which are effective in treating gastritis, flatulence, and irritable bowel syndrome.

Peppermint: Peppermint is an aromatic herb that calms the mind, soothes the nerves, and reduces headache pain. It's also used for nausea, depression, and anxiety, and can help uplift mood and dispel mental fatigue.

Lemon Balm: Lemon balm is a member of the mint family. Originating in Europe, it is well-known for its calming effect. It can be taken as an herbal tea and used for aromatherapy.

Hops: We tend to relate hops to beer, but it's also used as tea to relieve depression and calm the nervous system. Plus, it helps to alleviate other conditions often associated with stress, such as digestive disturbances.

Passionflower: Passionflower is one of the most popular herb teas sipped in Europe to relieve nervous tension, including insomnia, depression, and anxiety.

Valerian: Valerian has been used for generations. It's highly effective in calming stressed nerves. Its smell may take some getting used to, but once you reap the benefits, you may actually come to like it (or at least develop positive associations with it). If you find the odor too hard to take, try it in tablet or pill form. It works just as well.

Oat Straw: Oat straw tea is an excellent antidote for depression and nervous exhaustion due to its ability to nourish and calm the nerves. It can be used to treat insomnia and eliminate headaches. Plus, oat straw is good for reducing eyestrain.

Step Seven: Take a Bath

Lots of people say they aren't interested in sitting in a tub of water and instead opt for showers. However, there are real health benefits to a good, long, warm bath. Not only does bathing provide an antidote to stress and tension, it can also detoxify, stimulate circulation, and boost your immune system

Deep Relaxation: The muscle release associated with a good, hot bath helps to reduce cramps and tension headaches, and improve muscle elasticity. The process is similar to a massage and beneficial for everyone from athletes to those who sit at a desk all day. When a hot bath is followed with gentle stretching, the benefits to your musculoskeletal system may help to maintain muscle position and equalize tension on your bones. Emotional Benefits: A good book or magazine while relaxing in the bath can take your mind off financial and emotional worries and give you a clearer head when you need to address these problems at a later time. Keep your bath time a period without interruption to help guarantee a break from your hectic life.

Perspiration Rules: Keep the water hot enough to induce a sweat. The process of perspiration removes toxins from the body. You may even notice that a regular bath routine reduces perspiration odor so you have less of a need for deodorants to control body odor. The heat of the water also kills many strains of bacteria and viruses, decreasing the number of colds and infections you may get throughout the year.

Lymph System Improvement: The circulation of the lymph system required for the sweating process helps create a free-flowing system to remove toxins, bacteria, and viruses from your body. As you read in a previous chapter, the lymph system is the system responsible for stimulating immune response. Hot baths help increase lymph drainage and improve health. Also, the increased blood circulation improves all bodily systems by increasing the rate of nourishing blood cells to damaged tissue. In addition, dead cells are removed from the body more quickly, increasing the ability to stay healthy and energetic.

Cautionary Note: If you have high or low blood pressure, a bath that's too hot may cause problems. Always cool down slowly after a hot bath. Allow the water to cool or add cold water slowly to return your body temperature and circulation to normal before getting out of the tub. If you have any questions about the safety of a hot bath based on your medical conditions, talk to your doctor.

Step Eight: Trust in Love

The Beatles were on track when they sang "All you need is love," especially when it comes to maintaining your health. Not the passionate throes of romantic love with all its stressful ups and downs, but instead, the deep ties of a committed relationship. When you feel a loving connection from any kind of loving relationships, like long-term romantic partnerships or enduring friendships, you'll be more likely to:

Ban the Blues: Studies link social isolation to higher rates of depression, while committed partnerships are responsible for a happier and longer life. Studies also show a good partnership contributes to a decline in poor habits such as heavy drinking and drug abuse.

Have Lower Blood Pressure: That's the conclusion of a study in the Annals of Behavioral Medicine. Researchers found happy couples had the best blood pressure. One caveat: Unhappily married participants fared far worse.

Reduce Anxiety: After all these years, you may day-dream about a new romance, but when it comes to anxiety, a loving and stable relationship wins the prize. Researchers at the State University of New York at Stony Brook used functional MRI (fMRI) scans to look at the brains of people in love. They compared passionate new couples with strongly connected long-term couples. According to the report presented at the Society of Neuroscience, in long-term relation-ships there was activation in the brain's area associated with bonding and less activation in the area that pro-duces anxiety.

Feel Less Pain: In a study of more than 127,000 adults, long-term couples were less likely to complain of headaches and back pain. And that's not all. When researchers subjected 16 married women to the threat of an electric shock, those women holding their hus-band's hand showed less response in the brain areas associated with stress.

Better Brain Health: The give-and-take of a rela-tionship may help ward off mental decline. A Swedish study reports living as a couple in midlife is linked to a lower risk for cognitive impairment (unusually poor memory and mental function) during old age. Other research shows that regular social interaction, such as getting together with friends, belonging to a club, or doing volunteer work, also helps maintain brain vitality.

Fewer Colds: Loving relationships may also give the immune system a boost. Researchers at Carnegie Mellon University found that couples who exhibit positive emotions toward one another are less likely to get sick after exposure to cold or flu viruses. The study, published in Psychosomatic Medicine, compared couples who were happy and calm with those who appeared anxious, hostile, or depressed.

Faster Healing: Can the power of a positive relationship even make flesh wounds heal faster? It looks that way. Researchers at Ohio State University Medical Center gave couples blister wounds. The wounds healed nearly twice as fast in partners who interacted warmly compared with those who demonstrated a lot of hostility toward each other. The study was published in the Archives of General Psychiatry.

Step Nine: Smile!

Bright smiles are all over the beauty pages, touting pearly whites as essential to good looks. But it turns out there's more to our smiles than just flashy whites. Psychologists say smiles send out a host of positive signals. Here's what a big grin can do for you:

Increases Trust: Participants in one study reported to be 10 percent more likely to trust another person if they were smiling.

Boosts Forgiveness: Research shows we're more lenient with people who have broken the rules if they smile after their misdeed. It doesn't matter whether it's a false smile, a miserable smile, or a real smile, they all work to make us want to give the transgressor a break.

Helps Recover from Social Blips: Did you forget to buy your partner an anniversary present? Has someone's name slipped your mind? Embarrassed smiles also involve looking down. This combination elicits empathy from other people and studies show they'll think less of the slip and forgive us more quickly.

Helps Heal Hurt: Smiling is one way to reduce the distress caused by an upsetting situation. Psychologists call this the facial feedback hypothesis. And guess what? Forcing a smile even when we don't feel like it is enough to lift our mood slightly.

Gives Insight: Smiling makes us feel good, which also increases our attention and our ability to think holistically. When this idea was tested by social scientists, the results showed that participants who smiled performed better on tasks that required seeing the whole forest rather than just the trees.

Heightens Attraction: One study examined how men approach women in bars. When a woman only established eye contact with a man, she was approached 20 percent of the time. When the same woman added a smile, she was approached 60 percent of the time.

Adds Years: People who smile more may live longer. A study of pictures taken of baseball players in 1952 suggest those smiling outlived their nonsmiling counterparts by seven years.

Step Ten: Create a To-Do List

We all know the problems of having pages of things to do and no time to do them. Most of us are also aware that writing things down does not necessarily mean that we'll get them done. Still, there are real advantages to keeping a to-do list. But make sure that the important, goal-related activities are quickly scheduled into your planner, and not left on your to-do list. Also, limit your list to no more than five items.

Here are the real reasons to keep a daily list:

Supports Your Memory: When you list things that must be done, they're not forgotten. Our memory's ability is usually overestimated.

Clears the Mind for Other Things: Trying to mentally keep track of several items makes it harder to concentrates on a task at hand.

Relieves Anxiety: There's always the nagging fear that we may forget to do something. Writing it down relieves us of this anxiety.

Helps to Plan Ahead: The process of thinking about what has to be done keeps us proactive.

Helps Budget Time: Seeing everything that has to be done allows us to prioritize and allocate the most time to the more important tasks. Not having a to-do list leaves us vulnerable to spending too much time on trivial items.

Step Eleven: Read a Book

According to a Pew Research poll published in 2012, fewer people are reading than ever before. In fact, 19 percent of respondents said they hadn't read a single book (either electronic or print) over the previous 12 months. Those who love books already know the joys of reading—how it enriches our inner life and feeds our minds and imaginations. But reading offers a host of other benefits you might not have considered. Read on:

Relieves Stress: Removing oneself from a tense day by escaping into a fictional world has been shown to lower blood pressure.

Improves Concentration: Following the printed word in a book requires focus for a longer period of concentration than reading e-mails, magazine articles, or Web postings does.

Bumps Up Vocabulary: Remember in elementary school when you learned how to infer the meaning of one word by reading the context of the other words in the sentence? You get the same benefit from book reading.

Enhances Creativity: When you expose yourself to new ideas and information, your mind opens to fresh creative avenues.

Helps Sleep Patterns: If you make reading a habit before bed, a book acts as a kind of alarm for the body and sends the signal that it's time to sleep.

Builds Self-Esteem: When we're better informed we feel better about ourselves. Become an "expert" and people will come to you for answers. What an ego boost.

Improves Memory: Studies show if you don't use your memory, you lose it. Reading helps you stretch your "memory muscles" in a similar way. Reading requires remembering details, facts, and figures, and in literature, plot lines, themes, and characters.

Changes Your Life: Sometimes a book can be transformative and put you on a different path. (Maybe this is the one that does it!) You might decide to delve into a new hobby, pursue a different job, look at relationships differently, or follow through on a health or fitness plan. And that's the point about reading: It opens your world.

See How Far You've Come

Now that you've got the eleven steps down, you're ready to move on and discover some deeper truths about yourself. Take these two quizzes and uncover what's really behind the way you view your life. Then read the analysis and get suggestions on ways you can tune into your natural power.

Test One: Do You Have All the Energy You Need?

Studies show more than 10 percent of us have the feeling of disabling fatigue at any given time, and almost 65 percent of Americans say we just don't have the energy we need. But everyone has a unique EQ

(Energy Quotient): a combination of emotional balance, physical well-being, and healthy relationships. In order to truly be at your optimum energy level, you need to take care of all three essentials in your life.

In one hour the heart produces enough energy to raise a 1-ton weight 36 feet above the ground.

This test will help you to discover what *you* need to boost *your* EQ.

1. You're spending the weekend in a secluded cabin nestled beside a lake in the forest. You pack:

   a. Hiking boots and a swimsuit.

   b. A journal and lots of film.

   c. Your cell phone and laptop.

2. When the alarm rings you:

   a. Lie awake making a mental list of activities for the day.

   b. Rise immediately, wondering what the day will bring.

   c. Press the snooze button and pull the covers over your head.

3. For your birthday you'd rather have:

   a. A surprise party thrown in your honor.

   b. Dinner in your favorite restaurant with a loved one.

   c. Amnesia.

4. At the end of a working day, you feel:

   a. A little beat but ultimately satisfied with your accomplishments.

   b. Glad that you can start really living.

   c. Exhausted and desperate to relax.

5. Which of these statements sounds most like you?

   a. When I'm feeling distressed, I talk it over with a friend or loved one.

   b. Often I feel apprehensive or irritable, and I just don't know why.

   c. I refuse to let myself feel down.

6. When grocery shopping, does your cart have a higher proportion of:

   a. Fruits and veggies.

   b. Convenience foods like frozen entrées.

   c. Cookies and ice cream.

6. Do you drink water:

   a. Whenever you feel thirsty.

   b. To meet the recommended quota of eight 8-ounce glasses per day.

   c. Not often enough.

7. Which of these activities most appeals to you:

   a. Swimming.

   b. Sailing.

   c. Snoozing.

8. Choose the Saturday afternoon closest to your ideal:

   a. Taking a long walk or working out at the gym.

   b. Spending time with friends or family.

   c. Just hanging out with nothing on your plate.

9. Do you stay up late when there's something you want to watch on TV, even if you're tired?:

   a. Rarely.

   b. Sometimes.

   c. Frequently.

10. Do you mostly crave:
    a. Protein.

    b. Complex carbohydrates.

    c. Sugar.

11. When it comes to multivitamins, you take one:
    a. Daily.

    b. Sometimes, if you're feeling run-down.

    c. Never.

12. You usually keep your daily schedule:
    a. Partly booked but with some empty spaces.

    b. Flexible, to change with your mood.

    c. Sacred. Your never break plans.

13. You feel you're most rested after how many hours of sleep?
    a. 6 or fewer.

    b. 6 to 8.

    c. 9 or more.

Mostly A's: You Have Higher Energy Than Most

A spinning top with sparks of energy flying in every direction, you can keep going without taking a break.

You join the approximately 20 percent of the American population who falls into the category of type-A personality, with a naturally speedy metabolism and upbeat attitude that keeps you surging ahead. Although it's terrific that you've got energy-plus, everyone needs to rebalance once in a while. Here's what you need to concentrate on how to moderate your energy so you can keep going without burning out:

- ⬆ Get enough shut-eye. Although you might need less sleep than most, try to get to bed at the same time each night and awake the same time in the morning. Research shows everyone (even you!) needs at least 7 hours of sleep to function efficiently.

- ⬆ Take a vitamin B complex supplement. This stress-reducing vitamin keeps your energy humming.

- ⬆ Cut down on caffeine—you don't need it! Limit yourself to one cup a day. Try soothing herbal teas instead.

Mostly B's: You're Rock Steady

Since moderation is your motto, you try to pace yourself. To others it might appear that your accomplishments are effortless, but that's just because you can tame tough problems without wasting valuable energy. This comes naturally to you because your metabolism, adrenal glands, and body type are all set to release energy moderately and without radical highs or lows. But there are rare occasions when even you get stressed out. Recognize the signs—exhaustion, headaches, backaches, short temper, or sleeplessness. That's when it's time for you to relax and try these proven rejuvenation techniques:

- ⬆ Acupinch: Apply slight pressure and rub your outer ear with your thumb and first finger. This ancient acupressure point is a prime meridian for relaxing muscle tension from the body.

- ⬆ Breathe deeply for 60 seconds and watch your breath. This technique sends oxygen to your brain cells, giving your mood and thinking power a boost.

- ⬆ Take a catnap. Studies show just a 10-minute afternoon snooze can be as beneficial as an hour's worth of extra sleep.

Mostly C's: Your Energy Could Use a Boost

Soaking in a warm bath or snoozing on the couch is your idea of heaven, and it's a healthy practice to set aside time to relax. But if you have too little get-up-and-go, it's hard to get stuff done and meet your goals—which in turn can trigger the blues. It's a cycle. Low energy leads to sadness and sadness leads to low energy. Other factors? A lag in energy can be caused by a low-protein diet, lack of fresh air and light, or too little exercise. Whatever the underlying causes, here are simple energy-boosting techniques designed to match your natural EQ:

- ⬆ Perform Sun Salutations three times and get the benefits of mood-boosting light and exercise. You can do these simple yoga stretches in front of a window or outside. Go to the following website for more information on Sun Salutations at: http://www.wikihow.com/Do-the-Sun-Salute

- ⬆ Take a walk. Studies show just 20 minutes a day outdoors can speed your metabolism and uplift your mood.

- ⬆ Feel your feelings. When stressful situations arise, be authentic with your feelings: Let go of blame and keep your attention on what feels good.

- ⬆ Put it in writing. According to a University of California study, subjects who kept a daily gratitude journal rated 75 percent higher on scales measuring happiness and reported feeling revitalized and full of energy.

Test Two: Discover Your Personal Antidote to Stress

While most of us claim to hate stress, some of us actually need it as a mechanism to keep moving forward. In fact, the latest research shows up to 70 percent of us are biologically programmed to benefit from stress as long as we know how to deal with it in an effective way. Since a warm bath or exercising isn't for everyone, take this quiz to discover what works best to tame your tension.

1. While on the job, I'm more apt to:
    a. Welcome interruptions.

    b. Allow for interruptions, but don't really enjoy them.

    c. Let others know in advance I prefer not to be interrupted.

2. My idea of comfort dining is:
    a. Anything delivered.

    b. Something sweet and gooey.

    c. A three-course meal served in a restaurant.

3. When I feel the sniffles coming on, I'm more likely to:

    a. Ignore it and carry on.

    b. Take an over-the-counter remedy.

    c. Cuddle up on the couch, keeping tissues and hot tea within reach.

4. If I'm channel surfing, I'll likely stop on a:

    a. Reality show or the news.

    b. Crime or medical drama.

    c. Classic movie or sitcom.

5. My dream vacation would be a:

    a. Whirlwind five-city tour of Europe.

    b. Cross-country trip in fully equipped RV.

    c. Relaxing week at a slow-paced beach resort.

6. While driving along the highway, you'll find me putting my pedal to the metal in the:

    a. Fast lane.

    b. Middle Lane.

    c. Slow lane.

7. During my last lunch hour on a hectic work day, I:

   a. Happily ate at my desk.

   b. Got out for a short breather.

   c. Took the full hour off; I needed a break.

8. Which meal would you prepare for guests?

   a. A risky dish I've never tried before but is guaranteed to make an impression.

   b. Something complicated that I've already mastered.

   c. A simple tried-and-true menu I'm sure everyone will enjoy.

9. I would prefer to celebrate my birthday:

   a. With a big bash that was a total surprise.

   b. A well-planned get-together shared with my loved ones.

   c. An intimate dinner with a person I adore.

Mostly A's: You Crave Challenges

You enjoy the rush of the last minute and the race to the finish line, and with a schedule as packed as yours, it may seem like good news that you're a master at rushing around, multitasking, and waiting until the last second to tackle big projects. But when you play beat-the-clock and don't budget your time, you're bound to feel stressed out by the end of the day. Here are tension tamers tailored just for you:

- Set doable daily goals. The longer your list, the less likely you are to accomplish it and the more stressed-out you'll feel.

- Learn to take a breather and relax. Hyper-schedulers like you often view downtime as wasted time. It's not. Ask yourself: "What's really important in my life?" This simple question can help you set important priorities.

- Shut down distractions and limit multitasking. Studies show when you don't give full attention to a primary task, you'll make 30 percent more mistakes and can spend up to 20 percent more time correcting them.

- Schedule in pleasure. Stress junkies have a hard time sitting still, so recharge by making fun-packed dates with friends and family.

Mostly B's: You Keep a Balance

You've learned the secret to keeping stress in balance by looking at the big picture and not allowing yourself to get caught up in nit-picking details. It's all about setting priorities, feeling guilt-free when you do take time for yourself, and making sure your expectations aren't on overdrive. For the most part, you're already on the right track. Here are ways to stay moving on Easy Street:

- Delegate. Allow others who have expertise to carry some of the load. If it makes you uncomfortable to let someone else share responsibility, it's okay to check in once in a while.

- Open your palms. Surprisingly, a study shows this simple gesture of letting go actually helps release the impulse to take over situations.

- Eat foods rich in vitamin B6, which will help to keep your nervous system steady during up-and-down times: spinach, tuna, walnuts, white meat chicken and turkey, bananas, and raisins are all good choices.

- Have plan B ready. Psychologists say being prepared for change is the best way to prevent stress around it. When writing out your to-do list, pencil in alternatives.

Mostly C's: You're Ultra-Chill

Here's the good news: Stress-related illnesses like headaches, insomnia, and stomach ailments aren't on your horizon because you focus on the activity at hand, not just the result. You get pleasure from whatever you're doing. The downside? You're so easygoing that chores and responsibilities can mount up until you finally can't help but feel overwhelmed. It can be a messy house, a stack of unpaid bills, or clutter on your desk. Try these tips for living stress-free:

- ⬆ Create a special place for everything and put things away before they get out of hand.

- ⬆ Make a list of actions or goals you need to reach and then give yourself a deadline to achieve them. When you take actions step-by-step, you'll be less likely to feel overwhelmed.

- ⬆ Say "yes" instead of "no." Your first reaction may be to turn down a challenge, but think it over again. Exploring different options can actually expand your ability to cope.

- ⬆ Try tai chi, yoga, or meditation. You have the perfect personality for these proven stress-relieving practices. Plus, each of them can help you learn to stay focused as well as calm.

Last Word

Don't stop here. Allow yourself to experience a strong sense of accomplishment and pride knowing you've come so far. Perhaps just a few weeks ago, boosting your metabolism, detoxing, and looking to be happier and living a less-stressed life wouldn't have even crossed your mind.

Now give thanks that you've discovered ways to make your life better. Part of achieving goals is gaining the knowledge that you really can take control of your day-to-day experiences, and this gives new meaning to how you live your life.

Job well done! Congratulations!

If you don't like something, change it. If you can't change it, change your attitude.
~ Maya Angelou

Index

Acknowledgments

Gratitude to editor extraordinaire, Katherine Furman, Ulysses, Lauren Harrison, all my loyal friends, deep yoga buddies, loving neighbors, and to Brooklyn Roast, the most welcoming café for writers in all of Brooklyn—maybe the world.

About the Author

Robin Westen received an Emmy Award for the ABC health show *FYI*. She is currently the medical director for Thirdage.com, the largest health site for baby boomers on the Web. She is the author of *Ten Days to Detox*, the *Harvard Medical School Guide Getting Your Child to Eat (Almost) Anything*, as well as *V is for Vagina*, which is coauthored with Alyssa Dweck, MD. She's written feature articles for dozens of national magazines including *Glamour*, *Vegetarian Times*, *Psychology Today*, *SELF*, *Cosmopolitan*, and others. Robin has been practicing yoga, meditation, and cleansing for over fifteen years. She divides her time between Brooklyn and Vermont.